RATIONAL
MEDICAL
DECISION
MAKING

A CASE-BASED APPROACH

NOTICE

Medicine is an ever-changing science. As new research and clinical experience broaden our knowledge, changes in treatment and drug therapy are required. The author and the publisher of this work have checked with sources believed to be reliable in their efforts to provide information that is complete and generally in accord with the standards accepted at the time of publication. However, in view of the possibility of human error or changes in medical sciences, neither the author nor the publisher nor any other party who has been involved in the preparation or publication of this work warrants that the information contained herein is in every respect accurate or complete, and they disclaim all responsibility for any errors or omissions or for the results obtained from use of the information contained in this work. Readers are encouraged to confirm the information contained herein with other sources. For example, and in particular, readers are advised to check the product information sheet included in the package of each drug they plan to administer to be certain that the information contained in this work is accurate and that changes have not been made in the recommended dose or in the contraindications for administration. This recommendation is of particular importance in connection with new or infrequently used drugs.

RATIONAL MEDICAL DECISION MAKING

A CASE-BASED APPROACH

Goutham Rao, MD

Associate Professor
University of Pittsburgh School of Medicine
Faculty member, UPMC St. Margaret Family Medicine Residency and
  Faculty Development Fellowship Programs

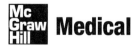 **Medical**

New York / Chicago / San Francisco / Lisbon / London / Madrid / Mexico
City / Milan / New Delhi / San Juan / Seoul / Singapore / Sydney / Toronto

Rational Medical Decision Making:
A Case-Based Approach

1 2 3 4 5 6 7 8 9 0   DOC/DOC   0 9 8 7 6

ISBN-13: 978-0-07-146397-3
ISBN-10: 0-07-146397-6

This book was set in Palatino by Techbooks.
The editors were James F. Shanahan, Maya Barahona,
and Peter J. Boyle.
The production supervisor was Sherri Souffrance.
Project management was provided by Techbooks.
RR Donnelley was the printer and binder.
This book is printed on acid-free paper.

Library of Congress Cataloging-in-Publication Data

Rao, Goutham.
    Rational medical decision making / Goutham Rao.—1st ed.
        p. ; cm.
    Includes bibliographical references and index.
    ISBN-13: 978-0-07-146397-3 (pbk. : alk. paper)
    ISBN-10: 0-07-146397-6 (pbk. : alk. paper)
1. Medicine—Decision making.   I. Title.
    [DNLM: 1. Decision Making.   2. Diagnostic Techniques
and Procedures.   3. Clinical Medicine—methods.
4. Research—methods.   5. Treatment Outcome.
WB 141 R215r 2007]
R723.5.R365 2007
610—dc22

                                        2006028014

Dedicated to a great statistician, teacher, and father
Professor U.L. Gouranga Rao
1936–2005

Contents

Preface

There are few professions that change quite as rapidly as medicine. A lawyer must keep abreast of new precedents and important cases. A teacher must become familiar with new standards and curricula. A businessman or businesswoman must keep a watchful eye on the competition. The way these professionals carry out their daily affairs, however, has not changed that much. Furthermore, the settings in which they work—the courtroom, classroom, or boardroom—have been largely unchanged. By contrast, even in the relatively short time since my graduation from McGill Medical School in 1993, the practice of medicine has changed dramatically.

As a physician, I have witnessed the rise and dominance of managed care in the United States and the public backlash that followed. Like most physicians, for several years, I prescribed hormone-replacement therapy to women entering menopause, but made a more recent frantic effort to get my patients to discontinue its use in light of new evidence suggesting it is harmful. Major threats to public health, with which all physicians should be familiar, have emerged over the past decade, including avian influenza and child obesity. New medicines and technologies have emerged so rapidly that the treatment of some illnesses today bears little resemblance to treatment only a few years ago.

How does a physician cope with the pace of change? Although change makes practicing challenging, many of the skills and attributes that made a good physician a hundred years ago are still important today: A good physician is empathic, communicates well, learns from experience, and is dedicated to his or her profession and patients. Practicing medicine is not and has never been a technical exercise. William Osler, that most famous of "McGill men," wrote:

> The practice of medicine is an art, not a trade; a calling, not a business; a calling in which your heart will be exercised equally with your head. Often the best part of your work will have nothing to do with potions and powders, but with the exercise of an influence of the strong

upon the weak, of the righteous upon the wicked, of the wise upon the foolish.[1]

Medicine remains an art and a calling, but the pace of change requires new skills that have become extremely important. New medical information comes primarily from original research. Original research is of variable quality and its applicability to the care of patients is often difficult to discern. Furthermore, research uses methodologies with which many physicians are unfamiliar and its results are expressed quantitatively in ways many physicians do not understand. To cope effectively with the pace of change, a physician or physician-in-training must have some understanding of how new information is generated and how best to interpret it. This book's purpose is to provide you with the basic skills you need.

I wish to acknowledge the following individuals for their extremely helpful suggestions and their careful reviews of the manuscript:

Jaspreet Brar, MD, MPH, Pittsburgh, Pennsylvania
Jill Landsbaugh, PhD, Pittsburgh, Pennsylvania
Kiame Mahaniah, MD, Lawrence, Massachusetts
Henry Wang, MD, MPH, Pittsburgh, Pennsylvania

---

[1] Osler W. *The Master Word in Medicine Aequanimitas.* Philadelphia: Blakiston and Son; 1904, p. 386.

RATIONAL
MEDICAL
DECISION
MAKING

A CASE-BASED APPROACH

Introduction

Origins of This Book

In the summer of 2001, I was asked to assume the role of course director of a mandatory course entitled *Clinical Epidemiology and Biostatistics* for all first-year medical students at the University of Pittsburgh. The course had been taught for several years by a physician with training in epidemiology, and for several years before him by a Ph.D.-trained epidemiologist. My predecessors were knowledgeable and skilled teachers. The course, however, was extremely unpopular with medical students. It followed the format of many introductory "traditional"epidemiology courses in which basic epidemiological terms and the features of different study designs are discussed. I took such a course in medical school some 10 years earlier and did not find it especially helpful. What was lacking was the relevance of epidemiological and statistical concepts to the practice of medicine. Explaining not only how research is carried out but also why it is important to understand how many clinical research studies are designed makes the subject more meaningful for medical students. One of the best ways to illustrate the relevance of epidemiology and statistics to physicians or physicians-in-training is with illustrative cases.

Between 2001 and 2003, I gradually redesigned *Clinical Epidemiology and Biostatistics* to better reflect content that medical students would find both more useful and interesting. The course was retitled *Introduction to Medical Decision Making*. Its goal was explicitly to help medical students become skilled interpreters of original medical research literature and to encourage application of the knowledge acquired through interpretation to the care of individual patients in a rational way. I envisioned that a medical student successfully completing the course would be able to find an original research article that addressed a question important to the care of an individual patient, convey a thorough understanding of the research methodology (including the statistical methodology), provide an accurate interpretation of the key results, and describe how such an article could influence clinical practice. In order to do that, a medical student at the very least needs to understand the basic format of most research articles, different study designs, and common statistics used in analyzing results. Given limited time, the course emphasizes only on what medical students are most likely to encounter in the medical literature.

In determining the content for Introduction to Medical Decision Making, I started by surveying the content of other courses with similar goals in medical schools in North America and Europe. Some medical schools still offer courses in epidemiology that follow a traditional format. Some schools offer courses in pure "bio" or "medical" statistics. Many schools offer experiences in "evidence-based medicine" (EBM), which emphasize the accurate assessment of the quality and practical interpretation of research evidence—an exercise known as "critical appraisal." Courses that emphasize this approach often ask students to meet regularly in groups to discuss the quality of new research articles. The "journal clubs" have been around in one form or another for decades. Introduction to Medical Decision Making borrows heavily from all these types of courses. The format and content of this book is largely based on this course.

Content of This Book

The content for this book includes information that is essential for physicians or physicians-in-training to interpret original medical literature accurately and efficiently. The chapter on biostatistics, for example, includes some basic statistical concepts and principles together with a description of common statistical tests of significance and how they are used.

With the exception of the first two chapters, the book is organized very similarly to a series of articles entitled the Users' Guides to the Medical Literature[1] published in the *Journal of the American Medical Association* in the early 1990s. This series established the foundation of EBM. Its purpose was to promote the identification, assessment, and application of the best available evidence to the care of patients. The users' guides are organized according to the overall purpose of different types of articles. For example, there is a users' guide entitled *How to Use an Article About Therapy or Prevention*. Although the structure of this book is similar to the organization of the users' guides and to other resources about EBM, the specific content differs in a couple of important ways. First, the authors of the users' guides state, "We don't attempt a course in research methods; the series is about using, not doing, research."[2] While the users' guides are a practical resource for using original articles, it is my belief that having some understanding of how research is designed promotes a greater understanding of how it should be applied. Aspects of research design, therefore, are discussed in some detail throughout this book.

The focus of most EBM resources is *critical appraisal*—determining whether the results of an original research article are valid (i.e., likely to represent the truth) and deciding how to apply the results to the care of patients. Throughout this book you will find information that can be used to determine the validity of research articles. Critical appraisal is not, however, discussed separately from aspects of the design and interpretation of studies. The Evidence-Based Medicine Working Group provides easy-to-use critical appraisal worksheets for different types of articles. Using the appropriate worksheet, it takes just a few minutes to determine whether a particular research article is valid and how to use its results. I have deliberately excluded these or other "quick" tools from the book. Since their introduction roughly 15 years ago, critical appraisal worksheets of various types have been used widely in journal clubs, as part of courses in EBM, and in clinical practice to assess new medical information. Indeed, in many cases, critical appraisal by using worksheets has become a substitute for learning biostatistics and principles of research methodology. There is nothing wrong with this. Critical appraisal worksheets, like EBM in general, were developed to be simple, practical ways for busy clinicians to interpret and apply new evidence. This book goes into greater detail partly to get readers interested in medical research of different types and partly because a deeper understanding of research papers makes determining the quality of a research article straightforward and obvious. A critical appraisal worksheet is not required.

This book deals only with original research in which some type of numerical or *quantitative* measure is used to describe outcomes (e.g., treatment A was associated with 34% reduction in the incidence of heart disease compared to treatment B). *Qualitative* research is extremely important though less commonly encountered and makes use of methods that are quite different from quantitative research. You can learn more about qualitative research by consulting references listed in the bibliography.

Original Research Articles

Original research refers to new contributions to the scientific literature. An original research paper has four important characteristics[3]: The paper's author(s) describe(s) a hypothesis (a term that will be discussed later) and a purpose for the study. The methods used to carry out the research are described in detail. The results of the research are also reported in detail. Finally, the researchers provide an interpretation of the results and their possible implications. The four characteristics are incorporated into four very distinct components that make up the format of most original research papers.

The *introduction* of an original research paper normally includes the general "context" of the study. For example, in a paper about a study of asthma, you might find information about how many children are affected by asthma and how serious a problem it is. A description of relevant previous research should also be included, as well as lack of previous research in the specific area to be addressed by the paper. Finally, the introduction should include the precisely defined purpose of the paper. Let us say we have a fictional paper about a new therapy for asthma that is more effective and easier to use than currently available treatments. The following could be a simple introduction.

> *Asthma is a serious disease that affects a large number of American children. Currently available treatments are expensive, not always effective, and difficult to use. Our new therapy is less expensive, more effective and easier to use than current treatments. It has not, however, yet been systematically evaluated. The purpose of this study is to evaluate the effectiveness and safety of our new treatment.*

The *methods* section of an original research paper includes a detailed description of how the research was carried out. Specifically, the type of study design, the type of subjects studied, the test or experimental procedures, how data was collected, how outcomes were measured, and the statistical methods used to analyze data should be included. Ideally, the methods should be described in enough detail for someone else to replicate the research and obtain similar results.

The *results* section of original research papers provides a summary of the findings of the research methods. In addition to text, results are often presented in the form of tables and figures.

Finally, the *discussion* section of an original research paper has several important purposes. It should link the results of the paper with the purpose as stated in the introduction. In other words, the discussion should explain how the results address the purpose. Also included in the discussion is a comparison of the results to previous studies with the same or similar purpose. The discussion should point out limitations of the study in terms of purpose, methods, and results. It should also suggest future directions for research in the same area. Finally, when possible, the discussion should provide recommendations for clinical practice.

Clinical research is the type of research which as a physician or physician-in-training you are most likely to encounter and find useful. Clinical research can be defined as the study of actual human patients or the records of actual human patients or theoretical models that deal primarily with patient care or decisions that affect patients directly.[4] This type of research has the most immediate impact upon patient care and is the focus of this book.

Finding Original Research

Sometimes you will simply "stumble upon" an original research paper that is relevant to your clinical practice or interesting to you for other reasons and is, therefore, worth reading and interpreting accurately. More often, questions are likely to arise during the course of patient care or during discussions in classes, lectures, or seminars, the answers to which are either unavailable from colleagues or textbooks. Answers to such questions can often be found in original research articles. For many years, the best way to find relevant original research articles has been by searching electronic databases such as Medline. Medline is widely available in different forms in most universities and hospitals. The National Library of Medicine provides a free, web-based version of Medline available from www.pubmed.com.

For several years, learning to search Medline systematically has been promoted as an important skill. Detailed instructions on how to search Medline can be found elsewhere.[5] Haynes et al. have developed tools for searching Medline that make use of the EBM paradigm for classifying original research articles.[6] Collectively, these tools are known as *clinical queries*.[7] Clinical queries allow you to find articles of a specific type without using formal rules or strategies to search Medline directly. Figure I.1 shows the main web interface for clinical queries that allows searching by clinical study category.

In addition to the aforementioned categories, clinical queries also allow you to search for systematic reviews, a type of original research paper that is discussed in this book. Consider this example: Let us say you are looking

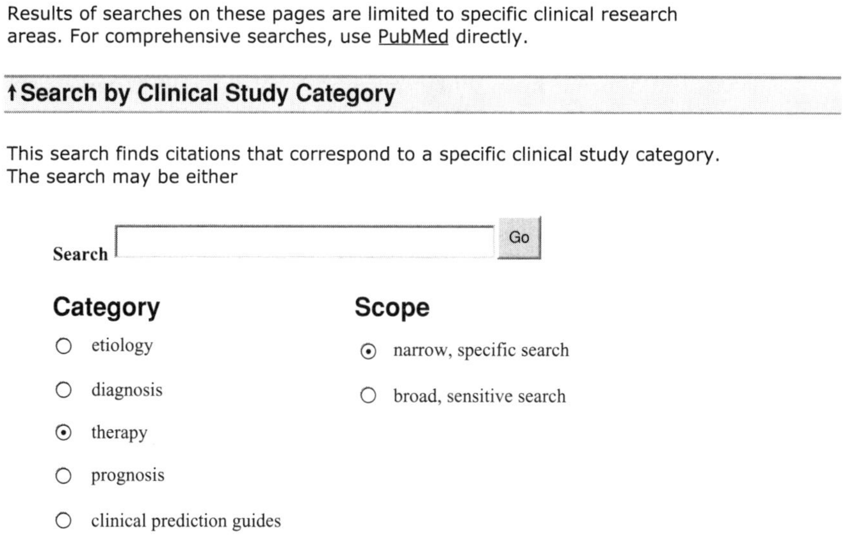

Results of searches on these pages are limited to specific clinical research areas. For comprehensive searches, use PubMed directly.

↑ Search by Clinical Study Category

This search finds citations that correspond to a specific clinical study category. The search may be either

Search [   ] Go

Category

○ etiology

○ diagnosis

◉ therapy

○ prognosis

○ clinical prediction guides

Scope

◉ narrow, specific search

○ broad, sensitive search

FIGURE I.1 PubMed Clinical Queries

(Reproduced from National Center for Biotechnology Information. Available from: /www.ncbi. nlm.nih.gov/entrez/query/static/clinical.shtml. Accessed April 11, 2006.)

for original papers that address treatment for sarcoidosis, a disease that affects the lungs and other organs. Punching in sarcoidosis and checking the buttons for therapy, and narrow, specific search, yields approximately 30 citations that deal specifically with the treatment of sarcoidosis. By clicking broad, sensitive search instead, you will get more than 3000 citations. These include not only articles specifically about treatment of sarcoidosis, but also articles about conditions similar to or mistaken for sarcoidosis, articles in which treatment of sarcoidosis may be discussed though not in depth, etc. Clinical queries is not perfect. You may find citations of articles that are not relevant to what you are looking for and the search strategies upon which clinical queries is based may on occasion miss articles that are very relevant. Nevertheless, clinical queries is an extremely valuable tool. It is less cumbersome than searching Medline directly. I recommend that you use it whenever you need to search for original research.

References

1. Users' guides to the medical literature. Available from: www.shef.ac.uk/ scharr/ir/userg.html. Accessed January 20, 2006.
2. Oxman A, Sackett DL, Guyatt GH. Users' guides to the medical literature. I. How to get started. *JAMA* 1993;270(17):2093–2095.
3. University of North Florida Library. What is original research? Available from: www.unf.edu/library/guides/originalresearch.html. Accessed January 20, 2006.
4. Merenstein JH, Rao G, D'amico F. Clinical research in family medicine: Quantity and quality of published articles. *Fam Med* 2003;35(4):284–288.
5. National Library of Medicine. Pubmed Tutorial. Available from: www.nlm. nih.gov/bsd/disted/pubmed.html. Accessed January 20, 2006.
6. National Library of Medicine. Summary of enhancements for clinical queries for MEDLINE for studies. Available from: www.nlm.nih.gov/pubs/ techbull/jf04/cq_info.html. Accessed January 20, 2006.
7. National Library of Medicine. PubMed Clinical Queries. Available from: www.ncbi.nlm.nih.gov/entrez/query/static/clinical.shtml. Accessed January 20, 2006.

A Brief History Lesson

O B J E C T I V E S

After reviewing this chapter, you should be able to accomplish the following:

1. In general terms, describe the origins of the modern medical journal.
2. Define evidence-based medicine.
3. Describe why evidence-based medicine developed.

1.1 Origins of the Modern Medical Journal

This book is about interpreting medical evidence, most of which is published in medical journals such as the *New England Journal of Medicine,* the *Journal of the American Medical Association*, the *Lancet*, and the *British Medical Journal*. Today's leading medical journals are venerable institutions that have disseminated the latest developments for generations and have had an enormous impact upon the way medicine is practiced around the world. Medical journals developed out of humankind's natural curiosity and desire to learn accompanied by a willingness to share the learning with others.

Medical journals, like all scientific journals, have their origins in early forms of the newspaper. When and where newspapers began is controversial. In ancient Rome, the *Acta Diurna* was a daily record of government decrees, news from wars, and results of athletic contests, which was posted in public places. In the Eastern world, the *Peking Gazette* was a newspaper founded in the seventh century AD. The earliest publication that we today would unmistakably recognize as a newspaper was the *Mercurius Gallo-belgicus*, which published European news in Cologne between 1588 and 1594. The establishment of newspapers in Europe was an extremely important development. Prior to newspapers, it was possible to announce important events in single issue "newsletters." The newspaper, however, could be counted on to supply the latest news, no matter how mundane. The idea of a reliable, regularly updated source of new information was born and is one of two major developments that was instrumental in the development of medical journals.

The second major development in the emergence of medical journals was the establishment of scientific societies. Proceedings of meetings of scientific societies, such as *L'Academie des Sciences* (France), the *Royal Society* (England), and *Academia del Lincei* (Italy), would be disseminated on a regular basis in a form similar to modern journals. Indeed, the first English scientific journal of any kind was the *Philosophical Transactions of the Royal Society.* When such societies were established in the sixteenth and seventeenth centuries, distinct disciplines of science, such as physics, chemistry, biology, and medicine, were only beginning to be recognized, and the first journals published articles that covered the entire breadth of the science of the day. The *Journal des scavans*, founded in Paris in 1665 by de Sallo, is generally acknowledged to be the first scientific journal. Its stated purpose was to

> *catalogue and give useful information on books published in Europe and to summarize their works, to make known experiments in physics, chemistry and anatomy that may serve to explain natural phenomena, to describe useful or curious inventions or machines and to record meteorological data, to cite the principal decisions of civil and religious courts and censures of universities, to transmit to readers all current events worthy of the curiosity of men.*

Today no journal, as you can imagine, has such a broad mandate. The *Philosophical Transactions of the Royal Society* and numerous other journals emerged soon afterward, particularly in Germany.

The oldest scientific journal devoted to medicine that is still in existence is Britain's *The Lancet*. It was founded by Thomas Wakley (1795–1862) in 1823 in London. Wakley, a qualified surgeon, originally founded *The Lancet* as a platform for political reform of the medical profession. Wakley was a firebrand and a radical whose scathing commentaries in the journal made him many enemies. A passage from his biography provides a glimpse of what his life was like:

> *Within six months after his marriage his home was broken up, his house burnt to the ground, his health temporarily impaired, his practice well-nigh destroyed, his reputation gravely impugned and the slanders that were rife about him were as widespread as they were malignant.*[1]

Wakley's house was destroyed by a gang following a rumor that he was involved in the executions of some of the gang's members. The rumor turned out to be false. Despite these and other troubles, *The Lancet* survived and thrived and is today recognized as among the most highly respected medical journals in the world.

1.2 Growth in Medical Literature

Since the founding of *The Lancet*, the number of scientific papers published in medical journals around the world has grown exponentially. The total number of medical articles is absolutely staggering. Much of the growth has taken place over the past 30 years as the pace at which new advances in medicine arrived has accelerated. Between 1978 and 1985, an average of 272,344 articles were published annually and listed in Medline—the electronic database that includes the vast majority of articles published worldwide. Between 1986 and 1993, this number had grown to 344,303 articles per year. Between 1994 and 2001, it had grown again to 398,778 articles per year.[2] The amount of biomedical knowledge contained in journals is doubling at a rate of roughly once every 19 years. A physician practicing general medicine today would have to read 17 articles a day, 365 days a year to keep abreast with the latest developments just in his field.[3] Needless to say, given that a physician's professional life is about a lot more than reading, this is impossible.

1.3 Evidence-Based Medicine

The idea that the decisions physicians make about the care of patients should be based on high-quality information from original research studies seems both obvious and uncontroversial. Unfortunately, many decisions physicians make in the practice setting are not based upon a careful or systematic review of the available evidence. There are several reasons for this. One reason has already been discussed: The sheer volume of new literature makes it impossible to keep abreast with important new developments. For this reason, busy physicians often make decisions based upon their own experience with patients or recommendations of colleagues. Second, there are many circumstances in usual clinical practice where important questions arise, but there is little or no evidence available to address it.

Evidence-based medicine, often abbreviated EBM, is a movement that arose over the past 20 years as a way of promoting the use of research evidence in the care of patients. David Sackett, one of the founders of the modern EBM movement, defines it more specifically as the "conscientious and judicious use of current best evidence from clinical care research in the management of individual patients."[3] The proponents of EBM have developed tools to help physicians identify, select, and analyze evidence for the care of patients. EBM is not, and was never meant to be, a substitute for other skills and resources used in practice. There is nothing wrong, for example, for physicians to make some decisions based only upon their own clinical experience, especially when scientific evidence is lacking. EBM is meant to complement, not replace, clinical experience.

As you might imagine, people began promoting the need to pay more attention to the evidence from research in the care of patients long before the term *evidence-based medicine* was coined. The idea that conclusions about natural phenomena should be based upon facts and observations rather than myth, superstition, or conjecture is an inherent part of the *scientific method*, which has been around in various forms since ancient times. According to the scientific method, scientists use observations and reasoning to propose tentative explanations of natural phenomena. These tentative explanations are known as *hypotheses*. They then test these hypotheses by conducting experiments. The experiments are designed such that it is possible for the hypothesis to be proven either true or false. Data from the experiments are carefully collected and analyzed. The experiments must be *reproducible*, meaning that if they are repeated in exactly the same fashion, one would obtain the same results. Once a hypothesis is supported through experiments, it is considered to be a *theory* and new predictions are based upon it.

Consider the following example: A physician from a bygone era notices that individuals in a certain part of a town seem to suffer much more often from dysentery. He visits that part of town and makes careful observations about its people, homes, streets, etc. He then compares these observations with those from another part of town where dysentery is uncommon. He notices that in the dysentery-prone district, drinking water comes from a canal in which raw sewage is disposed of. He formulates the hypothesis that water contaminated by raw sewage causes dysentery. He designs an experiment where 50 healthy volunteers are asked to obtain their drinking water for a period of 1 month from the dysentery-prone section and 50 others are asked to obtain their drinking water from a section that has been free of dysentery. The 50 people assigned to the dysentery-prone section develop dysentery at a very high rate, while others remain dysentery free. The physician concludes that the people who actually live in the dysentery-prone district are not especially susceptible to the disease but it is their water supply that makes them ill. He now proposes the theory that water contaminated with sewage causes dysentery. He predicts that separating sewage drains from drinking water will lead to fewer cases of dysentery. This project is completed by the local health authority and civil works authority. The physician's prediction turns out to be true.

The application of the scientific method has led to an enormous number of advances in medicine for hundreds if not thousands of years. The practice of bloodletting (an attempt to cure illness, especially fever, by cutting the skin or blood vessels) was never supported by "good" evidence. Nevertheless, it continued until the nineteenth century. Those who questioned the practice sought and obtained evidence to demonstrate that it was not only useless in curing disease but in many cases also very harmful. Among them was a military surgeon named Alexander Lesassier Hamilton who reported the results of an experiment conducted in Portugal in 1809. With two other surgeons, Hamilton sought to determine the impact of bloodletting compared to "caring for the sick" without blood-letting. He wrote

> *it had been so arranged, that this number was admitted, alternately, in such a manner that each of us had one third of the whole. The sick were indiscriminately received, and were attended as nearly as possible with the same care and accommodated with the same comforts. One third of the whole were soldiers of the 61st Regiment, the remainder of my own (the 42nd) Regiment. Neither Mr. Anderson nor I ever once employed the lancet. He lost two, I four cases; whilst out of the other third [treated with bloodletting by the third surgeon] thirty five patients died.*[4]

By the early twentieth century, carefully conducted experiments designed to evaluate the effectiveness of different therapies became common. The amount of evidence available to practicing physicians began to grow exponentially. The need to teach physicians how to use this evidence led to the modern EBM movement.

Key ideas of EBM were published in the 1990s as part of a series of articles titled Users' Guides to the Medical Literature in the *Journal of the American Medical Association*. The purpose of the series was to familiarize readers with the retrieval, analysis, and application of the best evidence. Unlike most textbooks of epidemiology which discuss research according to study design, EBM uses a paradigm for classifying the medical literature that is more practical for practicing physicians. The users' guides divide the medical literature according to subcategories that specify the key purpose or type of article. One of the users' guides, for example, is titled, "How to use an article about diagnosis."[5] Physicians considering adopting a new diagnostic test for their patients are likely to find a users' guide on diagnostic articles more useful than say, an epidemiological chapter on the design of cross-sectional studies, the research design often used to evaluate diagnostic tests. As noted in the Introduction, the EBM paradigm has been used as the organizational framework for chapters in this book.

References

1. Froggatt P, Snow J, Wakley T, The Lancet. *Anaesthesia* 2002;57:667–675.
2. Druss BG, Marcus SC. Growth and decentralization of the medical literature: implications for evidence-based medicine. *J Med Libr Assoc* 2005;93(4):499–501.
3. Sackett DL, Rosenberg WMC, Gray JAM, Haynes RB, Richardson WS. Evidence based medicine: what it is and what it isn't. *BMJ* 1996;312:71–72.

4. Claridge JA, Fabian TC. History and development of evidence-based medicine. *World J Surg* 2005;29:547–553.
5. Jaeschke R, Guyatt G, Sackett DL. Users' guides to the medical literature. III. How to use an article about a diagnostic test. A. Are the results of the study valid? Evidence-Based Medicine Working Group. *JAMA* 1994;271(5): 389–391.

Biostatistics for Medical Decision Makers

After reviewing this chapter, you should be able to accomplish the following:

1. List three reasons why it is important for physicians to have a basic understanding of biostatistics.
2. Provide examples of continuous and discrete quantitative data.
3. Provide examples of nominal and ordinal categorical data.
4. Given values from a small sample or population, calculate its mean and standard deviation.
5. List a minimum of three characteristics of a normal or Gaussian distribution.
6. Define z score.
7. Given a set of numbers, calculate its median.
8. Provide an intuitive explanation for the concept of degrees of freedom.
9. List the three components of the central limit theorem.
10. Explain the general principle of identifying differences among groups of observations.
11. Given a small number of groups of observations, each with a small number of values, perform an analysis of variance to determine if the groups are drawn from the same underlying population or not.
12. List the three assumptions upon which analysis of variance is based.
13. For each of the following statistical tests
    (a) describe the circumstances in which it should be used and its limitations;
    (b) describe the basic rationale underlying its calculations;
    (c) given a small, appropriate set of data, calculate the test statistic;
    (d) given a value of each test statistic and the data to which it corresponds, provide an accurate interpretation.
        t test
        Chi-square test
        Fisher exact test
        Mann–Whitney rank sum test
        Wilcoxan signed-rank test
        Kruskall–Wallis test

14. Rank a small set of observations so that the ranks can be used in calculating rank test statistics.
15. Describe the purpose of a "continuity correction."
16. In general terms, describe what is meant by "correlation."
17. Define coefficient of determination.
18. Determine the circumstances in which you would use Pearson's correlation coefficient and the Spearman rank correlation coefficient, and calculate and interpret the values of each for a small set of data.
19. Describe the purpose of regression.
20. List and describe three different types of regression.
21. Provide an accurate interpretation of the results of a regression analysis.

2.1 Introduction

Statistics is taught in many medical schools usually in the form of brief courses. Unfortunately, the subject is generally unpopular among medical students. The reasons are understandable. First, basic science courses in anatomy, physiology, biochemistry, molecular biology, and genetics as well as clinical courses that emphasize the diagnosis and treatment of disease dominate undergraduate medical curricula. The relevance of this material to the practice of medicine is obvious to most students. Statistics, on the other hand, seems out of place. Second, with the widespread availability of powerful statistical software packages and the expertise of statisticians, at least in most academic medical environments, the need to understand statistics, either for the interpretation or carrying out of research, seems questionable. Third, medical students approach statistics with trepidation. Much of what is taught in medical school requires only memorization and recall of facts. Even the most basic statistical concepts and calculations, however, require some skills in algebra and the ability to think abstractly. For many medical students, it has been several years since they exercised these skills. They are not accustomed to performing mathematical calculations. Most biostatistics textbooks are not a welcome alternative to formal courses. Unfortunately, medical students find most textbooks lengthy and intimidating. A majority of these books assume that readers have a considerable mathematical background and are accustomed to using it regularly.

There are several reasons why a basic understanding of statistics is important for physicians. Although the soundness of statistical methods and analyses in most medical research papers has improved in recent years, errors in methodology and analysis are still frequent, even in respectable journals. One reason is that peer reviewers of biomedical research articles feel comfortable providing a critique of the clinical or biological aspects of an article submitted for publication, but gloss over the statistics with which they are often unfamiliar. A basic understanding of statistics, therefore, helps a consumer of medical literature catch errors that may be critical to interpretation. Second, statistics is not as entirely irrelevant to everyday clinical practice as many people believe. Reports published by authoritative organizations in the United States and elsewhere over the past few years have emphasized that clinical care often does not meet basic quality standards. Practicing physicians have come under increased pressure both to meet standards and also to carefully and regularly assess the quality of care they provide. The value of this type of self-directed "audit" is enhanced by a little understanding of statistics. Finally, a significant proportion of medical school graduates will incorporate basic science or clinical research or other scholarly activity into their careers. These activities will undoubtedly at some point require use of statistics for the design of studies or the analysis of data. Statisticians in academic medical environments are typically overwhelmed, and their help is not always available. Complex statistical issues will always require their help, but some knowledge of statistics provides physician-researchers with a degree of independence.

What exactly is biostatistics? A simple definition is the application of statistics to the fields of medicine, biology, or related disciplines. The field is broad and complex. Just about everything in this book could be encompassed under the umbrella of biostatistics. Chapter 3, for example, introduces you to the likelihood ratio, a measure of the usefulness of diagnostic tests. Although included in the section on "diagnostic reasoning," there is no question that the likelihood ratio is a type of "statistic." In the context of this book, biostatistics refers to terms and concepts that are useful specifically for (1) understanding the statistical procedures and analyses found in most research papers and (2) performing calculations and analyses to better understand simple, quantitative information. The emphasis in this chapter is only on what basic statistical skills a physician needs to know to practice medicine or interpret scientific information. Many biostatistical concepts, therefore, are not included. Others are deliberately not covered in depth. The goal is to equip you with the basics of biostatistics as one part of the set of skills needed to care for patients. The content is designed to answer two basic questions about key statistical concepts and tests: (1) What precisely are their definitions? (2) What is the basic idea behind them? Keep in mind that though rational medical decision making requires some biostatistics, biostatistics by itself is not enough to make rational medical decisions.

2.2 Types of Data Encountered by Physicians

Biostatistics deals with data, and a simple way to begin to learn about statistics is to review the types of data you are likely to encounter. Biostatistical data comes in two basic forms. *Quantitative* data refers to measurements or *variables* (measurements that vary from person to person, time to time, etc.) to which a specific quantity or numerical value can be assigned. For example, a patient's systolic blood pressure can be measured as 130 mm Hg. An elderly patient may experience an average of three episodes of dizziness a week. These are two forms of quantitative data but there is an important distinction between them. Blood pressure, unlike the number of episodes of dizziness per week, can take any value within a biologically plausible range. For example, a patient's systolic blood pressure could be 131, 93, or 132.5 mm Hg (though blood pressure is seldom measured so precisely). A patient's hemoglobin level can be 12.3, 13.5, or 9.35 mg/dL. Quantitative variables that can take any value within a plausible range are called *continuous*. Body weight and height are two additional examples. On the other hand, the number of episodes of dizziness per week, the number of patients a physician sees per hour, or the number of adults in a household are all variables that cannot take on any value within a given range. It is possible to see 4 patients an hour, but not 4.5. These types of quantitative variables are sometimes called *discrete*.

Data also comes in the form of categories. Sex, for example, is a *categorical* variable to which only two categories (male or female) can be assigned. Such categorical variables with only two possible values are called *binary*. Similarly, a person's astrological sign can only assume one of 12 *named* values. These are called *nominal* data (data to which a name is assigned). The other type of categorical data includes categories which can be placed in a logical *order* (i.e., *ordinal*). Systolic blood pressure can be categorized as optimal, high-normal, stage 1 hypertension, and stage 2 hypertension. These categories are more than just names. Stage 2 hypertension is much worse than optimal blood pressure. The categories can therefore be placed in order from lowest to highest. Similarly, a headache can be described as mildly painful, moderately painful, or extremely painful.

We will deal with both types of quantitative and categorical data throughout this text.

2.3 Summarizing Data with Descriptive Statistics

CASE 2.1

Hatchett Lake is a tiny community with a total population of only 100 inhabitants. The mayor is concerned about contamination of local soil and the water supply by lead. He asks you to measure the blood lead levels of all residents in the town. After obtaining the data, how would you summarize the results?

There are several ways to summarize this data. Blood lead levels are measured on a continuous scale. To create an easy-to-digest visual display of the data, one can divide the plausible range of values of blood lead into intervals and record the frequency of observations in each interval. The resulting graph is known as *histogram.* The histogram of blood lead levels is shown in Figure 2.1.

This visual display gives us some idea of the range of values of blood lead. Some simple numerical data is also very useful. The familiar "average," known as the *mean* value, is easy to calculate. It is simply the sum of values divided by the number of values. Mathematically,

$$\mu = \Sigma X/N,$$

where μ denotes the mean of a population, Σ means "sum of," and X represents each value in the population. Therefore, ΣX is the sum of all the values in the population. N is the number of values in the population. In Hatchett Lake, μ (blood lead) is therefore $\Sigma X/100$. It happens to be 2.5 μg/dL.

The mean is an extremely useful summary statistic. It is known as a measure of *central tendency.* A population with a mean blood lead of 7.5 μg/dL is likely to be quite different from a population with a mean blood lead of 2.5 μg/dL. The mean, however, tells us nothing about the *variability* of the values in a population. Consider the populations of three blood lead levels on the next page.

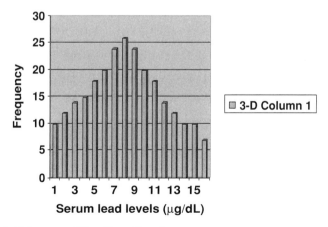

FIGURE 2.1 Histogram of Blood Lead Levels

Population A (Set A)	Population B (Set B)
2, 17, 38 μg/dL	17, 22, 18 μg/dL

The mean of each of these sets of data is 19. However, set B is quite different from set A. In set B, all three values are closely clustered around 19. In set A, by contrast, the three values are quite far apart from each other. There is more *variability* in set A compared to set B. We can quantify this variability precisely by determining by how much on the average, each value in each set deviates from its mean. Consider set A. The first value deviates from the mean of 19 by $(2 - 19)$ or -17. The second value deviates from the mean by $(17 - 19)$ or -2. The third value deviates from the mean by $(38 - 19)$ or 19. We could simply add up these deviations and divide by the number of observations in the set to obtain an average deviation, a measure of the set's variability. The problem is that two of the deviations are negative and one is positive. Adding them up and dividing by three gives us an average deviation of zero. This implies that there is no variability. Instead, we can square each deviation and divide by the number of members in the set. This quantity is known as the *variance* of the population. Mathematically,

$$\sigma^2 = \Sigma(X - \mu)^2 / N,$$

where σ^2 is the variance, $\Sigma(X - \mu)^2$ is the sum of the squared deviations of each value in the population set from the mean, and N, of course, is the number of members of the population. For set A, the variance is

$$\sigma^2 = \Sigma(2 - 19)^2 + (17 - 19)^2 + (38 - 19)^2 = 654/3 = 218.$$

For set B, the variance is

$$\sigma^2 = \Sigma(17 - 19)^2 + (22 - 19)^2 + (18 - 19)^2 = 14/3 = 4.7.$$

Clearly, the variance of set A is much greater than that of set B. The unit for these variances of blood lead levels is $(\mu g/dL)^2$. This is not the original unit in which blood lead is measured. To make the variances more useful, we take their square roots to return to the original units of μg/dL. This measure of variability (σ) is known as the *standard deviation*. Mathematically,

$$\sigma = \text{square root of the variance}$$

or

$$\sigma = \sqrt{\frac{\Sigma\left(X_i - \mu\right)^2}{N}}.$$

For set A, $\sigma = \sqrt{218}$ or approximately 14.8 μg/dL; for set B, $\sigma = \sqrt{4.7}$ or approximately 2.2 μg/dL. We can, therefore, describe set A as a population of three with mean blood lead level of 19 μg/dL and standard deviation of 14.8 μg/dL and set B as a population of three with a mean blood lead level of 19 μg/dL and standard deviation of 2.2 μg/dL.

Look carefully at the histogram (Fig. 2.1). It has a symmetric bell shape. There are some people in Hatchett Lake with very low blood lead levels and others with very high levels, but the largest number have levels clustered in the middle. This bell shaped curve is extremely common for many types of data and is known as a *normal* or *Gaussian* distribution (also known as a bell curve). Data are likely to be normally distributed when each value is dependent upon many, often small, random factors. Think of the things that may determine a person's blood lead level. The level may depend upon age, body composition, different aspects of body chemistry, where the person lives, nutrition, occupation, etc. The number of potential influences upon blood lead is very large. The same is true for other variables that are normally distributed, like height. Consider the heights of adult men in a community. Their heights depend upon different aspects of genetics, nutrition, ethnicity, chronic illness, etc. By contrast, variables that depend only upon a few, easily defined factors are not normally distributed. Imagine that your computer has broken down and you have decided to call a customer service hotline for help. The time you spend "on hold" before you receive help likely depends upon just a couple of factors, such as the time of the day and the number of technicians available to answer calls.

The normal distribution has some important and easy-to-understand statistical characteristics due to its symmetric shape. The mean value of data is found at the center or highest point of the curve (Fig. 2.2).

Regardless of the actual variables being measured or their values, if the data is normally distributed, approximately 34% of values will lie within 1 standard deviation on either side of the mean (or a total of 68% of values within 1 standard deviation on both sides of the mean). Roughly 47.7% of values lie within 2 standard deviations of the mean on either side (or roughly 95% for both sides), and 49.8% of values lie within 3 standard deviations of the mean on either side (or roughly 99.6% of values for both sides). Each distance of 1 standard deviation away from the mean is also called a z score. Therefore, 99.6% of all values lie within three z scores from the mean on either side. These properties are true for all normal distributions, regardless of their mean and standard deviation.

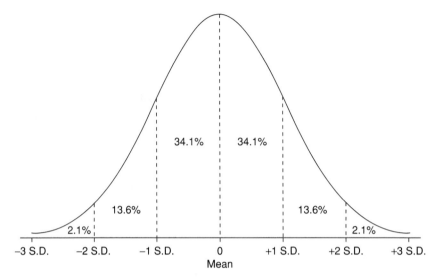

FIGURE 2.2 Normal Distribution

Since a value roughly 2 standard deviations above the mean is larger than 97.5% of all the values in the distribution, we can describe it as being at the *97.5th percentile.* Similarly, since the mean is larger than 50% of the values, the mean of a normal distribution is always at the 50th percentile. Percentiles, rather than number of standard deviations away from the mean, are a practical way to understand where a particular data point lies.

Fig. 2.3 shows the same normal distribution with percentile markings. As already mentioned, not all data is normally distributed. Consider the population of a wealthy seaside community, which for the sake of simplicity has only five inhabitants. The annual incomes of each of the residents are

$22,000,

$17,000,

$33,000,

$26,500, and

$12,500,000.

The mean income of the community is a staggering $2,519,700. In reality, it turns out that the first four members of the community work at the estate of the individual who earns $12,500,000 a year. Using the average of

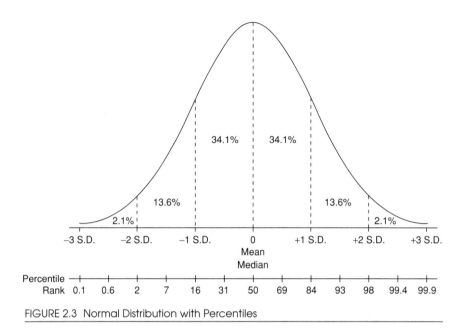

FIGURE 2.3 Normal Distribution with Percentiles

income to describe the community is misleading because the mean income is *skewed* upward by one individual. Skewed distributions do not have a symmetric shape around their means (see Fig. 2.4). An example is shown next. Instead of describing a skewed distribution using a mean, a better alternative is to use the *median*, the point that separates the lower and upper half of the values (i.e., the 50th percentile of values). The first step in finding the median is to number the values in order of magnitude. The median of any set of data is defined simply as the $(n+1)/2$ observation, where n is the total number of observations. For example, the median of the set of numbers 3, 6, 11, 16, 19, is the $(5+1)/2$ or 3rd observation. In this case, the corresponding value is 11. If a set of data contains an even rather than an odd number of values, the median is defined as the average of the $n/2$ and $(n/2)+1$ observations. For the set of data, 11, 15, 19, 20, 23, 35, the $n/2$

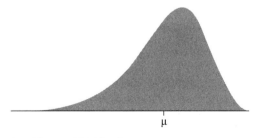

FIGURE 2.4 Example of Skewed Distribution

observation is 19. The $(n/2) + 1$ observation is 20. The median is therefore the average of 19 and 20 or 19.5. Just as the median is an alternative to the mean to describe a skewed distribution, the *interquartile range* is an alternative to the standard deviation to describe the variability of a skewed distribution. The interquartile range is simply the values corresponding to the 25th and 75th percentile of values. Let us assume that the seaside community described previously has 500 rather than 5 inhabitants and that there are 100 millionaires and 400 middle-class or low-income workers. One could describe this skewed population as having a median income of let us say, $28,000 with an interquartile range of say, $15,100–$52,000. This provides a reasonably meaningful description of incomes in the community.

2.4 Populations and Samples

A population is simply all the members of a particular group. All women age 40–49 in Seattle, WA, for example, constitute a specific population. Normally, it is not possible to study all members of a population. Consider trying to determine the average blood lead level of the population of all adults in the United States. This would be extremely difficult. As an alternative, we could simply study some American adults and use our results to draw conclusions about the entire population. The adults we choose to study would be a *sample* of the larger population. The use of samples to draw conclusions about a population is known as *statistical inference.*

There are many ways to obtain a sample. To determine the mean level of blood lead of American adults, for example, one could measure lead levels in all adults in one small neighborhood in Boston to draw conclusions about all American adults. The trouble is that adults in one small neighborhood in Boston may be quite different in important ways from adults in say, San Diego, CA. The adults in such a sample may not, therefore, be *representative* of all American adults. Researchers usually want samples that are representative of the population from which they were selected. One way to accomplish this is to obtain a *random sample.* Members of the population are selected at random to form the sample. Such samples have two important characteristics: First, each member of the population has an equal chance of being selected for the sample. Second, the choice of one member of the sample does not affect the choice of another member being chosen (i.e., the choices are *independent* of each other). Let us say we wish to obtain a random sample of 100 adult residents of Columbus, OH. We could use the Columbus phonebook and open it without looking 100 times to a particular page and then also without looking, select a name from the page at random. In theory, through this technique, each adult in Columbus has an equal likelihood of being selected for the sample. The choice of one adult for the sample does not influence the choice of another. In reality, random sampling is more complicated than this.

Just as one can describe a population with simple, descriptive statistics, the same can be done with samples. The mean of a sample is simply the sum of all its constituent values divided by the number of values. Mathematically,

$$\overline{X} = \Sigma x/n,$$

where $\overline{X}$ (read "x bar") is the symbol for the mean of a sample, rather than a population, x is the variable representing individual values, and n is the size of the sample.

The standard deviation of a sample is defined mathematically as follows.

$$S = \sqrt{\frac{\Sigma(X_i - \overline{X})^2}{n - 1}},$$

where S is the symbol for the standard deviation of a sample and $\Sigma(X_i - \overline{X})^2$ is the sum of the squared deviations away from the sample mean. Note that in order to get the variance of the sample, we divide this sum by $n - 1$ (the sample size $- 1$) rather than n. This $n - 1$ is known as the number of *degrees of freedom* and has been a source of bewilderment among students of statistics for generations. An explanation follows.

2.5 Degrees of Freedom

Why does the formula for the standard deviation use $n - 1$ rather than n? Mathematical explanations are quite complicated and frequently omitted even from statistics textbooks. A more intuitive explanation, which will be helpful later in this chapter as well, is sufficient for medical decision makers. The number of degrees of freedom is literally the number of values that are "free to vary" in a sample. We use samples to make estimates about populations. When we obtain statistics about samples, we use them as estimates of statistics about populations. Statistics about populations are called *population parameters.* Consider a town with a population of 10,000 families. We wish to estimate the mean and standard deviation of family income in the town. It would be cumbersome to collect this information from every family. Instead, we choose to obtain data from a random sample of 100 families. Let us say we calculate the mean income of these 100 families to be $32,000. We can therefore estimate that the mean family income in town is also $32,000. Since we know the mean family income estimated from our sample and the total number of families in our sample, it is easy to calculate the total income of all our families in the sample. We simply multiply $100 \times \$32,000$ to obtain $3,200,000. Now, let us say you know the sample size of 100, the mean income of $32,000, and 99 of the

100 values. Can you calculate the last value? Indeed, it is easy to calculate as $3,200,000 minus the sum of the other 99 values. The missing value is therefore fixed by knowledge of the mean and the other 99 values. It is not *free to vary*. By using our sample mean as an estimate of the population mean, we have *used up one degree of freedom*. In general, the number of degrees of freedom of a sample is one less than the total number of values in a sample.

This explanation describes why "degrees of freedom" are so-named. Using $n - 1$ in the formula for the standard deviation of a sample also serves a practical purpose. Intuitively, you can imagine that a random sample of 100 individuals from a population of 10,000 would have more variability than the whole population. This is because those 100 individuals could come from any part of the population distribution. Assuming the population is normally distributed, most individuals in the population come from the middle of the distribution. By dividing the sum of the squared deviations from the sample mean by $n - 1$ rather than n (i.e., to obtain the variance), we are arithmetically accounting for the fact that the sample standard deviation is bigger than that of the population from which it was drawn.

2.6 Samples for Estimation of Population Parameters

Let us return to our example of selecting samples of 100 from a town of 10,000 families to determine the mean and standard deviation of income in town. In the example in previous section, the mean of our sample of 100 was $32,000. If we were to obtain another sample of 100 from the same population, would its mean be exactly $32,000? It would almost certainly not. It is unlikely to contain the same composition of families. We could obtain a third sample which would be slightly different than the first two. Indeed, we could continue to obtain samples of 100 and get slightly different mean family incomes each time. There are millions of possible different samples of 100 that can be drawn from a population of 10,000. Let us assume that we obtain all possible samples of 100 and each time calculate the mean of each sample. We can then plot each of the means. The resulting plot has some very important properties (Fig. 2.5).

The plot of the means is approximately normally distributed. This distribution of means itself has a mean (i.e., the mean of the means) and standard deviation. The standard deviation of the distribution of means is known as the *standard error of the mean*. It is important to note that the plot of the means will always be normally distributed *even if the population from which the samples are drawn is not normally distributed*. Why? Recall that whenever the value of a variable is determined by a number of small, independent factors, it is likely to be normally distributed. In the case of the

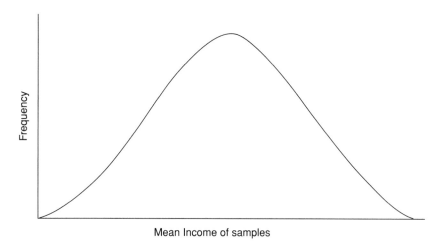

Mean Income of samples

FIGURE 2.5 Plot of Means of Samples

means of samples of 100 families, each data point is a mean that is determined by 100 different factors (i.e., the income of individual families). This
is why the means are normally distributed.

Normality of the distribution of the means of samples is one of three
components of what is known as the *central limit theorem*. The theorem consists of the following three statements:

- The distribution of sample means will be approximately normal regardless of whether the distribution of the original values in the population is normal or not.
- The mean of the means of all possible samples equals the population
  mean.
- The standard deviation of the distribution of the means of all samples
  (standard error of the mean) is equal to the standard deviation of the
  population divided by the square root of the sample size.

The proofs of the second and third statements are beyond the scope of
this text. Mathematically the third statement can be expressed as

$$\sigma_x = \sigma / \sqrt{n},$$

where σ_x is the standard error of the mean (or SEM), σ is the standard
deviation of the population, and n is the sample size. Note that the SEM
will always be smaller than the population standard deviation. This makes
sense because means "pull" data points together. A distribution of means,

therefore, has less variability than the distribution of values in the original population.

Why did we bother with this? Clearly, it is unlikely that we would ever obtain all possible samples from a population. Using the third statement of the central limit theorem, one can estimate the SEM *from a single sample* according to the formula

$$s_{\bar{x}} = s/\sqrt{n},$$

where s_x is the SEM estimated from a single sample, s is the standard deviation of the sample, and n is the size of the sample. We use the SEM estimated from a single sample as a measure of *uncertainty in the estimate of a mean of a population based upon a sample mean.* Let us say that we decide to obtain just one sample of 100 families to estimate the mean family income among the population of a town. We calculate the mean income in our sample to be $25,000 and the sample standard deviation to be $1000. The SEM is simply

$$s_{\bar{x}} = 1000/\sqrt{100} = \$100.$$

The SEM of our estimate of $25,000 as the mean family income of the town's population is $100. Note that this *is not the standard deviation of the family income in the town.* It is an estimate of the precision of our sample mean as an estimate of the population mean. The standard deviation of family income in the town would likely be much larger than $100. As sample size increases, the precision of our sample mean as an estimate also increases. If we obtain a sample of 1000, for example, then

$$s_{\bar{x}} = 1000/\sqrt{1000} = \$32.$$

2.7 Basic Principles of Identifying Differences Between Groups

One of the most common uses of statistics in the medical literature is to test for significant differences among groups of observations. Typically, a new treatment is compared in some way to one or more existing treatments (called *controls*). Many physicians find the statistical procedures used mysterious and are prone to accept the results of this type of statistical testing without either any scrutiny or understanding. It is true that many statistical tests are very complicated. All rely, however, on a few simple principles. Understanding basic principles makes it much easier to understand the complexities of statistical tests in general and makes them seem less intimidating.

CASE 2.2

Your friend Jack recently invented a new diet drug he calls "Meltaway-Rx." He also evaluated this new drug in a study comparing it to two older drugs, A and B, among three groups of five patients. Table 2.1 lists the weight loss results for all 15 patients.

TABLE 2.1   Weight Loss in 3 Months (kg)

Drug A	Drug B	Meltaway-Rx
2	6	8
3	8	9
10	4	3
2	2	10
8	10	5

Is Meltaway-Rx better than the older drugs?

One obvious way to begin to answer this question would be to calculate the mean weight loss associated with each drug. For drug A, the mean is $(2 + 3 + 10 + 2 + 8)/5 = 5$ kg; for drug B, the mean is $(6 + 8 + 4 + 2 + 10)/5 = 6$ kg; for Meltaway-Rx, the mean is $(8 + 9 + 3 + 10 + 5)/5 = 7$ kg. According to the mean weight loss, therefore, Meltaway-Rx is the best drug. If only life were so simple!

The complicating factor is individual variation in the response to each drug. For example, among patients treated with drug B, why did one patient lose 2 kg and another 10 kg? The patient who lost 10 kg may be different in some fundamental ways. He or she may, perhaps have a body chemistry that is more responsive to drug B. After all, this patient lost as much as anybody on drug A or on Meltaway-Rx. The reasons why one patient loses more than another are innumerable. Essentially, such differences are *unexplainable*. Comparing groups involves measuring this unexplainable variation and comparing it to the variation we can explain.

Look carefully at the data in Case 2.2 (Table 2.1). We know that the three groups differ with respect to their mean weight loss. This could be because each group receives a different treatment, or simply because individuals in each group respond differently to different drugs. We, therefore, have two explanations for the differences among the three groups. Differences due to the effect of being in a particular group are *explainable* (since the explanation is the fact that the three treatments are different). We can compare the explained to the unexplained variation (variation within each group due to individual differences). What if the explained variation is much bigger than the unexplained variation? This means that the effect of being in a particular group is much larger than the individual differences within each group. We would conclude that the three drugs have different effects. On the other hand, if the three drugs had the same effect on weight loss, we would likely find that the explained variation is no bigger or smaller than the unexplained variation. This illustrates the fundamental principle that underlies all statistical tests comparing groups (known as *tests of significance*). All tests of significance are a ratio of explained variation/unexplained variation.

When this ratio is large, we conclude that groups are different; when it is small, we conclude that they are not. Statisticians use dozens of different tests of significance depending upon the type of data and groups they are dealing with. I will discuss a few of the more common tests later. For the time being, knowing that as complicated as statistical calculations can get, the purpose is to calculate the simple ratio, should be comforting.

2.8 Analysis of Variance

To determine the ratio of explained/unexplained variation (or variability), we will now complete a procedure known as an *analysis of variance* (ANOVA). ANOVA is normally performed using statistical software. Few physicians will ever have the need to perform the procedure, let alone by hand. The purpose of this section is only to demonstrate how the ratio of explained/unexplained variability is obtained. Similar calculations are performed for a wide variety of tests of significance.

Let us return to the example of Case 2.2. To determine the explained and unexplained variability, we *partition the total variability*. The total variability in all three groups is calculated assuming that all observations in the three groups are part of one large group. We calculate the *total sum of squares* (SS_{total}). A sum of squares is like a variance except that the sum of squared differences between observations and the mean is not divided by n or $n - 1$. To calculate the SS_{total}, we use the mean of all the observations under study. This is known as the *grand mean*. SS_{total} is given by

$$SS_{total} = \Sigma(X_n - \text{grand mean})^2.$$

For Case 2.2, the grand mean is $[2 + 3 + 10 + 2 + 8 + 6 + 8 + 4 + 2 + 10 + 8 + 9 + 3 + 10 + 5]/15 = 6$.

$$SS_{total} = \Sigma(2 - 6)^2 + (3 - 6)^2 + \cdots = 140.$$

Next, we can calculate the explained variability. This is the variability explained by differences from group to group. We begin by calculating a quantity known as the *between groups sum of squares:*

$$SS_{\text{between groups}} = n\Sigma(\bar{x}_{\text{group}} - \text{grand mean})^2.$$

This $\bar{x}_{\text{group}}$ is the mean of each of the groups and n is the number of observations in each group (in this case, 5). Intuitively, it makes sense to multiply the sum of the squared deviations of each group mean from the grand mean by n, because these deviations apply to each member of each group. For Case 2.2,

$$SS_{\text{between groups}} = 5\Sigma(5 - 6)^2 + (6 - 6)^2 + (7 - 6)^2 = 10.$$

The unexplained variability is calculated using a quantity known as the *within groups sum of squares.* The squared deviations of each value from its corresponding group mean are added together:

$$SS_{\text{within groups}} = \Sigma(x_n - \bar{x}_{\text{group}})^2.$$

For Case 2.2,

$$\begin{aligned}
SS_{\text{within groups}} = {} & \Sigma[(2 - 5)^2 + (3 - 5)^2 + (10 - 5)^2 + (2 - 5)^2 + (8 - 5)^2] + \\
& [(6 - 6)^2 + (8 - 6)^2 + (4 - 6)^2 + (2 - 6)^2 + (10 - 6)^2] + \\
& [(8 - 7)^2 + (9 - 7)^2 + (3 - 7)^2 + (10 - 7)^2 + (5 - 7)^2] = 130.
\end{aligned}$$

This calculation is awfully cumbersome! It is easier to use the simple relationship,

$$SS_{\text{total}} = SS_{\text{between groups}} + SS_{\text{within groups}}$$

so,

$$SS_{\text{within groups}} = SS_{\text{total}} - SS_{\text{between groups}}$$

For Case 2.2,

$$SS_{\text{within groups}} = 140 - 10 = 130.$$

When we calculated the standard deviation of a sample, we divided the sum of squared deviations from the mean by the number of degrees of freedom. Similarly, we need to divide the between and within groups sums of squares by their corresponding number of degrees of freedom.

The total number of degrees of freedom is simply the total number of observations -1. For Case 2.2,

$$DF_{\text{total}} = 15 - 1 = 14.$$

The between groups degrees of freedom is simply the total number of groups -1. For Case 2.2,

$$DF_{\text{between groups}} = 3 - 1 = 2.$$

The within groups degrees of freedom is simply the number of groups multiplied by 1 less than the number of observations in each group (assuming the groups have an equal number of observations). For Case 2.2,

$$DF_{\text{within groups}} = 3 \times (5 - 1) = 12.$$

We can also use the following simple relationship:

$$DF_{\text{total}} = DF_{\text{between groups}} + DF_{\text{within groups}} \quad \text{or,}$$

$$DF_{\text{within groups}} = DF_{\text{total}} - DF_{\text{between groups}}.$$

The next step in our ANOVA is to divide the between and within groups SS by their corresponding degrees of freedom. The resulting quantities are called *mean squares* (MS) and are equivalent to variances.

$$MS_{\text{between groups}} = SS_{\text{between groups}} / DF_{\text{between groups}}$$

For Case 2.2,

$$MS_{\text{between groups}} = 10/2 = 5$$

and

$$MS_{\text{within groups}} = 130/12 = 10.8.$$

We now have two measures of variability. If the between groups MS is much larger than the within groups MS, this is evidence that the groups are indeed different from each other. We can calculate a statistic known as the *F ratio*:

$$F = MS_{\text{between groups}} / MS_{\text{within groups}}.$$

If F is very large, it is possible to conclude that the groups being compared are significantly different (i.e., the groups are samples of different populations). If F is close to or less than 1, it tells us that random variation or individual differences are greater than the effect of being in a particular group. We can conclude, therefore, that the groups are not significantly different (i.e., the groups all come from the same population).

How large is a large F? The F ratio itself has a distribution of values. Statisticians designate a large F as one that is as big as or bigger than 95% of the values in the distribution (known as a *critical value*). The F distribution also depends upon the number of between groups (numerator) and within groups (denominator) degrees of freedom. A table of F values is given in the Appendix (Table A.2). For Case 2.2, $F = 5/10.8 = 0.46$. The numerator degrees of freedom is 2. The denominator degrees of freedom is 12. The critical value of F from the F table is 3.8853. Our value of F is much smaller than this. We can conclude, therefore, that the three weight loss treatments are not significantly different in their effects.

We have completed an ANOVA. ANOVA requires three important assumptions that must be at least approximately true to draw valid conclusions:

1. Each sample (in Case 2.2, each group) is independent of the others and is randomly selected from the underlying populations. Knowing the values in one group tells us nothing about the other groups.

2. The populations from which the samples were drawn are normally distributed.

3. The variances of each population from which the groups are drawn are equal, though the means may or may not be different. In other words, the degree of variability in the underlying populations is the same. This assumption is known as *homogeneity of variance*.

If these assumptions are not even approximately true, ANOVA is inappropriate.

ANOVA and the F test are useful for illustrating how groups can be compared statistically to identify significant differences. The F test is not, however, among the most useful tests of significance. It tells us only that groups being compared are statistically different but does not tell us which groups differ from each other. Let us assume, for example, that we had obtained a large F in Case 2.2. It would not tell us if groups A and B were the same and differed from Meltaway-Rx, or if groups A and Meltaway-Rx were the same and differed from group B, or if groups B and Meltaway-Rx were the same and differed from group A. We will now discuss *some* of the most common statistical tests. The derivation of the formulae that follow is unnecessary for physicians. For each test, there are three fundamental things you should understand: First, they are all variations of the explained variation/unexplained variation ratio which use different approaches; second, the choice of test depends upon the type of data you are dealing with; and finally, the value that you obtain through calculations for each statistic is compared to a distribution of values derived with the assumption that there is no significant difference among the groups being compared.

2.9 t Test

One of the most common statistical procedures in medical research is the comparison of one group to one other. The t test is the most common test of significance performed when comparing the means of two samples of *continuous, normally distributed* data. The statistic t is given by t = difference in sample means/standard error of difference of sample means.

The difference in sample means is analogous to the explained variation (differences observed due to the effect of either treatment). This difference can be positive or negative. What matters is the relative magnitude of the difference rather than its sign. The standard error of the difference is analogous to unexplained variation. Case 2.3 illustrates the formula, calculation, and application of the t test.

CASE 2.3

Your friend Jack has developed a new blood pressure lowering medication, which he has compared to an older medication (hydrochlorothiazide) in a group of 10 patients, 5 of whom received each drug. He measured the number of millimeters of mercury drop in systolic blood pressure in each patient after 1 week on his or her assigned drug. The results are given in Table 2.2.

TABLE 2.2   Drop in Blood Pressure (mm Hg) After 1 Week

Hydrochlorothiazide	New Drug
10	25
5	20
15	15
5	15
20	10

Drops in blood pressure are measured on a continuous scale and are normally distributed.

Is Jack's new drug a superior blood pressure lowering agent to hydrochlorothiazide?

We can start by computing the means for each group. For hydrochlorothiazide, the mean drop in blood pressure is 11 mm Hg; for the new drug, the mean drop is 17 mm Hg. The difference is 6 mm Hg. This difference is the numerator in our formula for t. To determine the standard error of this difference, we rely on a mathematical principle, the proof for which you will find in many statistics textbooks.

The variance of a sum or difference of two randomly selected variables is simply the sum of the variances of the two populations. If A is a variable drawn from a population with variance σ_A^2 and B is a variable drawn from a population with variance σ_B^2, then the variance of all possible values of A + B or A − B is

$$\sigma_{(A+B)\,or\,(A-B)}^2 = \sigma_A^2 + \sigma_B^2.$$

This relationship is also true for variances computed from samples. If A and B are samples rather than populations, then

$$S_{(A+B)\,or\,(A-B)}^2 = S_A^2 + S_B^2.$$

The SEM is just a standard deviation of means. The relationship applies in this situation as well. Let us say we have two samples with means of $\overline{O}$ and $\overline{U}$. The variance (SEM squared) of a difference of the means is given by

$$(SEM)_{\overline{O}-\overline{U}}^2 = (SEM)_{\overline{O}}^2 + (SEM)_{\overline{U}}^2.$$

Taking square roots on both sides, we get

$$SEM_{\overline{O}-\overline{U}} = \sqrt{(SEM)_{\overline{O}}^2 + (SEM)_{\overline{U}}^2}.$$

So our equation for *t* is now

$$t = \frac{\overline{O} - \overline{U}}{\sqrt{(SEM)_{\overline{O}}^2 + (SEM)_{\overline{U}}^2}}.$$

Recall that $SEM = s/\sqrt{n}$, where n is the sample size. Our equation for *t* now becomes

$$t = \frac{\overline{O} - \overline{U}}{\sqrt{s_{\overline{O}}^2/n_{\overline{O}} + s_{\overline{U}}^2/n_{\overline{U}}}},$$

where $s_{\overline{O}}^2$ and $s_{\overline{U}}^2$ are the variances of the samples with mean $\overline{O}$ and $\overline{U}$, respectively, and $n_{\overline{O}}$ and $n_{\overline{U}}$ are the respective sample sizes. Recall that one of the basic principles of tests of significance is comparing the value of the test statistic to the value of test results obtained under the assumption that groups being compared are not significantly different, i.e., they come from the same population. If the hydrochlorothiazide and new drug samples come from the same population, then variances, $s_{\overline{O}}^2$ and $s_{\overline{U}}^2$, are both estimates of the same population variance. We can replace these two estimates of the population variance with a single estimate that is an average variance also known as the *pooled-variance* and designated s^2:

$$s^2 = \frac{(n_{\overline{O}} - 1)\, s_{\overline{O}}^2 + (n_{\overline{U}} - 1)\, s_{\overline{U}}^2}{n_{\overline{O}} + n_{\overline{U}} - 2}.$$

Our equation for t becomes

$$t = \frac{\overline{O} - \overline{U}}{\sqrt{s^2/n_{\overline{O}} + s^2/n_{\overline{U}}}}$$

Returning to Case 2.3, the difference in means is 6, $s_{\text{hydrochlorothiazide}}^2$ is 42.5, $s_{\text{new drug}}^2$ is 32.5, and n is 5 in both cases. Our pooled-variance is

$$s^2 = \frac{(4 \times 42.5) + (4 \times 32.5)}{8} = 37.5,$$

$$t = \frac{6}{\sqrt{(37.5/5 + 37.5/5)}} = 1.55.$$

Is this a big t? As in the case of F, we compare our value of t to a distribution of values obtained under the assumption that there are no significant differences between groups. Once again we need the number of degrees of freedom (v). The number of degrees of freedom is $2(n - 1)$ where n is the number of observations in each group. In Case 2.3, $2(n - 1)$ is 8. We now consult a table of t values (see Table A.3). We can decide that if our value of t lies within the extreme 5% of values (the probability of obtaining a value greater than the observed value of t is 5% or less), the two groups come from two separate populations and the new drug does have an effect. Looking at the t table under 8 degrees of freedom and $p = 0.05$, we obtain a critical value of 2.306. Our value is considerably less than this. We can conclude, therefore, that the new drug is no more effective than hydrochlorothiazide.

We have illustrated a basic application of the t test. There are actually several types of t tests. t tests can also be "one tailed" or "two tailed." In a two-tailed test, we are concerned whether the value of t we obtain exceeds extreme values in either tail of the t distribution. In a one-tailed test, we are only concerned whether our value of t exceeds extreme values in one tail. The critical values of t are lower for one-tailed tests. Two-tailed tests are almost always preferred. From the standpoint of practicing physicians, knowing what a t test is and the general approach to obtaining a value of t is sufficient. You can learn more about different types of t tests from most statistics textbooks.

2.10 Chi-Square Test

The chi-square (χ^2) test is used to test differences among groups of data measured on a *nominal* scale. Let us now consider Case 2.4.

CASE 2.4

Your friend Jack has just invented a new type of motorcycle helmet and wishes to test its effectiveness in preventing death among motorcyclists involved in accidents resulting in head injury. His data is presented in Table 2.3.

TABLE 2.3   Type of Helmet and Outcome from Accident

Type of Helmet	Survived Head Injury	Died	Total
New helmet	79	6	85
Old helmet	71	24	95
Total	150	30	180

It appears that Jack's helmet is superior to the old helmet in helping motorcyclists survive head injury. Is this actually true?

Table 2.3 is called a *contingency table*. It shows the relationship between two or more, usually categorical, variables. The table in Case 2.4 is a 2 × 2 table because there are two types of treatments being studied and two possible outcomes. Each of the four numbers in the 2 × 2 table (i.e., ignoring the totals) is said to occupy a *cell*. The χ^2 statistic is defined as follows.

$$\chi^2 = \Sigma\{(\text{observed}-\text{expected value of cell})^2/\text{expected value of cell}\}.$$

Once again, this ratio fits into our general concept of tests of significance as the ratio of explained/unexplained variation. The explained variation is what we observe due to different treatments. In this case, it is the difference between these observations and the expected values. What is the expected value of a cell? It is the value we would expect if the new treatment had no effect on surviving a head injury (i.e., the new helmet is no better than the old helmet). We do not have a precise explanation for what determines this rate of death (i.e., could be a number of different factors) and so the expected value represents unexplained variation. Among motorcyclists who wore the old helmet, 71/95 or 75% survived and 25% died. It is obvious from the table that the new helmet is associated with a higher survival rate. A total of 30 people (or 17%) died in this study. If the new helmet was no better than the old helmet, 17% of both the

TABLE 2.4   Expected Outcomes Assuming No Difference in Helmet-Type

Type of Helmet	Survived Head Injury	Died	Total
New helmet	71	14	85
Old helmet	79	16	95
Total	150	30	180

motorcyclists who wore the new and old helmets would have died. We can create a new table using these "expected values" (see Table 2.4).

We can now calculate χ^2 as

$$\chi^2 = \frac{(79-71)^2}{71} + \frac{(6-14)^2}{14} + \frac{(71-79)^2}{79} + \frac{(24-16)^2}{16}$$

$$= 10.29.$$

Like other tests of significance, χ^2 has a distribution of values under the assumption of no difference between the groups being compared that depends upon the number of degrees of freedom (v). This v for contingency tables like Table 2.4 is the number of rows -1 times the number columns -1, or

$$v = (r-1)(c-1).$$

For a 2 × 2 table, v is always $= 1$. We can compare our value of χ^2 to the distribution of values arranged in a χ^2 table (see Table A.4). Once again using a level of significance of $p = 0.05$, we find that the critical value of χ^2 for one degree of freedom is 3.841. Our value for the helmet experiment greatly exceeds this. Jack's helmet, therefore, is superior to the old helmet, which confirms our initial expectation based on simply looking at Table 2.3.

Unfortunately, statistics is often more complicated than one would like. A more accurate calculation of χ^2 when there is one degree of freedom (i.e., for 2 × 2 tables) is obtained using what is known as the *Yates correction*. The correction slightly reduces the value of χ^2 we calculate. The rationale for the correction is that the distribution with which we compare our calculation is a continuous curve along which χ^2 can take on any value. Our calculation using one degree of freedom, by contrast, can only take on certain discrete values. Using the Yates correction, χ^2 is given by

$$\chi^2 = \Sigma\{(|\text{observed value of cell} - \text{expected value of cell}| - 1/2)^2/ \text{expected value of cell}\}$$

The vertical line "|" is the symbol for absolute value (i.e., the magnitude of a number without its sign). Using this formula, χ^2 is approximately 9.03. This still exceeds our critical value of 3.841, and we still reach the same conclusion that Jack's helmet is superior.

2.11 Fisher Exact Test

The χ^2 test is not valid for 2×2 contingency tables with very small samples. Using the χ^2 test when any *expected* value in a cell is less than 5 is inappropriate. The reason is a little complicated but can be summarized as follows: The distribution of χ^2 for a 2×2 table follows a pattern known as a *binomial distribution*. The χ^2 test, however, relies upon an approximation known as the normal approximation to the binomial distribution, that is, a normal distribution can be used in place of a binomial distribution as an approximation. This approximation becomes invalid for small samples. The *Fisher exact test* is used instead.

CASE 2.5

Jack has completed a small study to test a new surgical technique to stop gastrointestinal ulcers from bleeding. He compared this new technique to an older "banding" procedure in a small group of patients. His results are shown in Table 2.5.

TABLE 2.5   Outcomes of New Technique Versus Banding

Technique Used	Bleeding Stopped	Continued Bleeding	Total
New technique	2	3	5
Banding	3	3	6
Total	5	6	11

Jack's new technique appears to be worse than banding. Is this result statistically significant?

The general form of a 2×2 contingency table used to perform the Fisher exact test is shown in Table 2.6.

TABLE 2.6   Algebraic Format for 2×2 Table

Treatment	Outcome 1	Outcome 2	Total
Treatment 1	A	B	R_1
Treatment 2	C	D	R_2
Total	S_1	S_2	N

The Rs and Ss stand for "rows" and "sums," respectively. The *exact* probability of obtaining any 2×2 table (*assuming there is no difference between treatments*) is given by the following formula:

$$P = \frac{R_1!R_2!S_1!S_2!}{N!a!b!c!d!},$$

where ! is the mathematical *factorial* function and means multiplying each value by successively smaller integers until you get to 1. For example, 5! is $5 \times 4 \times 3 \times 2 \times 1 = 120$. By convention, $0! = 1$.

The exact probability of Jack's table is therefore

$$P = \frac{5!6!5!6!}{11!2!3!3!3!} = 0.43.$$

The probability of obtaining Jack's results assuming that the two treatments are equivalent is, therefore, 0.43. We are also interested, however, in obtaining not only the exact probability of this result but also the probabilities of other results that may be less likely to occur, assuming that there is no difference between the two treatments. This is analogous to calculating the probability of an entire tail or tails of a continuous distribution. The tails consist of more than just one result. What results would be less likely than the one Jack obtained? Imagine that Jack's new surgical treatment was even worse than what was initially observed (i.e., it stopped bleeding in even fewer patients). We can construct two additional 2×2 tables by reducing the smallest element in our table by 1 and then calculating values for the other three cells *making sure that the row and column totals are constant* (see Tables 2.7 and 2.8).

TABLE 2.7   New Technique Stops Bleeding in 1 Fewer Patient

Technique Used	Bleeding Stopped	Continued Bleeding	Total
New technique	1	4	5
Banding	4	2	6
Total	5	6	11

TABLE 2.8   New Technique Stops Bleeding in 2 Fewer Patients

Technique Used	Bleeding Stopped	Continued Bleeding	Total
New technique	0	5	5
Banding	5	1	6
Total	5	6	11

The probabilities associated with each of these tables are the following:

$$p = 5!6!5!6!/11!1!4!4!2!2! = 0.08 \quad \text{(Table 2.7)}.$$

$$p = 5!6!5!6!/11!0!5!5!1! = 0.01 \quad \text{(Table 2.8)}.$$

Now let us assume that Jack's treatment is actually better than banding. Once again, keeping row and column totals constant, we can construct Tables 2.9–2.11.

The probabilities of Tables 2.9–2.11 are as follows:

Table 2.9, $p = \dfrac{5!6!5!6!}{11!3!2!2!4!} = 0.32;$

Table 2.10, $p = \dfrac{5!6!5!6!}{11!4!1!1!5!} = 0.06;$

Table 2.11, $p = \dfrac{5!6!5!6!}{11!5!0!0!6!} = 0.002.$

TABLE 2.9   New Technique Stops Bleeding in 1 Additional Patient

Technique Used	Bleeding Stopped	Continued Bleeding	Total
New technique	3	2	5
Banding	2	4	6
Total	5	6	11

TABLE 2.10   New Technique Stops Bleeding in 2 Additional Patients

Technique Used	Bleeding Stopped	Continued Bleeding	Total
New technique	4	1	5
Banding	1	5	6
Total	5	6	11

TABLE 2.11   New Technique Stops Bleeding in 3 Additional Patients

Technique Used	Bleeding Stopped	Continued Bleeding	Total
New technique	5	0	5
Banding	0	6	6
Total	5	6	11

These six probabilities represent the probabilities of getting Jack's result or a more extreme result (i.e., one that would occur with less probability), under the assumption that the two treatments are not different. To calculate the probability of getting Jack's result or a more extreme result we simply add the probability of getting Jack's result and the probabilities of the tables that are less likely to occur than Jack's result. In this case, the probabilities of all six tables should be added together.

$$p(\text{Jack's results or more extreme}) = 0.43 + 0.08 + 0.01$$
$$+ 0.32 + 0.06 + 0.002 = 0.90.$$

The probability of getting the results Jack obtained or more extreme results, *assuming there is no difference in the two treatments*, is 0.90. If we use p less than or equal to 0.05 as the point at which we would conclude the treatments are different, Jack's results clearly do not show that the two treatments are significantly different. We have completed the Fisher exact test. Notice that we considered both the possibilities that Jack's new procedure was even worse than observed, as well as the possibility that it was better than observed. In summing probabilities, we used probabilities that were less likely than the observed results in *either direction*. We have therefore performed a *two-tailed* Fisher exact test. For a one-tailed test, we would consider only the probability of the observed table and values of tables whereby Jack's new procedure was even worse than what was observed.

This example describes the general procedure for the Fisher exact test: When any element of a 2 × 2 contingency table is less than 5, calculate the exact probability of the table. Then, calculate the exact probabilities of all other tables that can be constructed keeping the row and column totals constant. Add the exact probability of the observed table to the probabilities of tables that are less likely (i.e., more extreme) to get the total probability of getting the observed result or more extreme results under the assumption that the treatments being compared are equal.

2.12 Rank Tests

ANOVA and the t test are valid only when the distributions of values being studied are normal or approximately normal. Recall that the calculations involved in ANOVA or the t test rely heavily upon means and standard deviations (or variances). ANOVA and the t test are called parametric tests because they are based on estimates of two population parameters (the mean and standard deviation) that define a normal distribution. Parametric tests are very useful because they allow us to draw conclusions about populations. If a distribution is not normal, one cannot rely upon the mean and standard deviation as accurate descriptors and therefore cannot use parametric tests.

One way of dealing with observations that are drawn from populations that are not normally distributed is with the use of ranks. Tests based on ranks are *nonparametric*. They are not as useful as parametric tests in drawing conclusions about populations. They are used when the data being studied is not normally distributed. They are also useful to test for differences in data that are *ordinal* rather than continuous. In fact, a rank itself is a type of ordinal scale. The idea of ranks or "ranking" is very simple.

Let us say we have three values of systolic blood pressure:

150 mm Hg

110 mm Hg

180 mm Hg

We can assign ranks to each of these values from smallest to largest as follows:

1. 110 mm Hg
2. 150 mm Hg
3. 180 mm Hg

When there is more than one observation with the same magnitude, the tied observations receive the average rank they would have received had they not been tied. Consider the following observations of blood pressure:

130 mm Hg

140 mm Hg

130 mm Hg

150 mm Hg

140 mm Hg

Notice that there are two values of 130 mm Hg and two of 140 mm Hg. Let us assume that there are no ties and rank them in order. We have

1. 130 mm Hg
2. 130 mm Hg
3. 140 mm Hg

4. 140 mm Hg

5. 150 mm Hg

Since it makes no sense to assign different ranks to values of the same magnitude, we use the average rank that tied values would have received had they not been tied. The average of ranks of one and two, for example, is 1.5. The average of ranks 3 and 4 is 3.5. Our final ranking is the following:

1.5. 130 mm Hg

1.5. 130 mm Hg

3.5. 140 mm Hg

3.5. 140 mm Hg

5. 150 mm Hg

Rank tests make use only of the ranks and not the original observations to determine if there are significant differences among groups.

CASE 2.6

Jack has developed a new version of an older diet drug. Table 2.12 shows the results of a small study he completed; in this table the new drug is compared to the old drug in terms of the number of kilograms of weight loss among five patients.

TABLE 2.12   Kg of Weight Loss Among Patients

New Drug	Old Drug
3	6
9	4
7	

Let us assume this data comes from populations that are not normally distributed. The mean weight loss with the new drug is $6\frac{1}{3}$ kg compared to 5 kg with the old drug. Is the new drug really superior?

We will answer this question using the *Mann–Whitney rank sum test*. In reality, of course, it would be unusual to have a study group with just two or three members and tests based on ranks are normally based on larger samples. Case 2.6 will be used only to explain the general principles of determining differences based on ranks. The first step is to rank the

TABLE 2.13   Weight Loss and Ranking of All Patients in Study

Observation (kg of Weight Loss)	Rank
3	1
4	2
6	3
7	4
9	5

observations in order of magnitude from smallest to largest regardless of whether they are in the new drug group or the old drug group. Tied observations are assigned a rank equal to the average of the ranks they would have been assigned had there not been a tie. Then we can revisit the table in Case 2.6 and show the data with its corresponding ranks (Tables 2.13 and 2.14).

We compare the ranks in the new drug and old drug groups. The basic rationale is the following: If the new drug was no better than the old drug, we would expect that the sum of the ranks in both groups would be roughly the same. In other words, each group would have its fair share of high ranks and low ranks and the totals for each group would not be too different. If on the other hand, one group was significantly different from the other, we would expect that high ranks would cluster in one group and the sum of the ranks in one group would be significantly higher than the other.

We need to calculate only the sum of the ranks in the smaller of our two samples (or in either one if the samples are the same size). This sum is the Mann–Whitney rank sum statistic T. For Case 2.6, $T = 3 + 2 = 5$. Is this a large value? Let us assume that the type of drug has no influence on weight loss and, therefore, the rank of observations is not related to the type of drug and is due only to *random or unexplained variation*. Two observations make up our smaller sample. Those two members, under these

TABLE 2.14   Weight Loss and Ranking by Type of Drug

New Drug		Old Drug	
Observation	Rank	Observation	Rank
3	1	6	3
9	5	4	2
7	4		

TABLE 2.15   Possible Rank Sums Assuming No Difference in Groups

1	2	3	4	5	Rank Sum (T)
X	X				3
X		X			4
X			X		5
X				X	6
	X	X			5
	X		X		6
	X			X	7
		X	X		7
		X		X	8
			X	X	9

circumstances, could assume any of the five possible ranks. The number of possible *unique* combinations of ranks and rank sums is quite small and easy to illustrate with a table (Table 2.15).

If the type of drug has no effect, any of these rank sums could occur at random. There are 10 rank sums. A rank sum of 5 is possible 2/10 or 20% of the time, as is a rank sum of 6 or 7. A rank sum of 4 is possible 1/10 or 10% of the time. Our most extreme rank sums are 3 and 9, which are possible 10% of the time, respectively. Our rank sum has a 20% chance of occurring alone. When combined with the more extreme rank sums of 3 and 9 (10% each), the total probability of obtaining a rank sum as extreme or more extreme than that observed is 40% assuming the two drugs have the same effect. It is safe to say, therefore, that there is insufficient evidence to conclude that the two drugs are different. This example illustrates the basic idea of comparing rank sums to all possible rank sums. It is artificial due to the very small number of observations. We cannot use our conventional level of significance of 0.05 to describe the 5% of most extreme rank sums of T, since each rank sum has at least 10% chance of occurring. With larger numbers of observations, T becomes more useful. If there were seven total observations, there would be 35 possible rank sums. The number of possible rank sums increases dramatically as the size of each sample increases. With larger samples, though T is a nonparametric statistic, its distribution does resemble a normal distribution with the following characteristics:

Its mean is given by

$$\mu_T = n_S(n_S + n_B + 1)/2,$$

where n_S is the size of the smaller group and n_B is the size of the larger group. Its standard deviation is given by

$$\sigma_T = \sqrt{n_S n_B (n_S + n_B + 1)/12}.$$

Using this mean and standard deviation, we can obtain the test statistic Z_T, which can be compared to the z scores corresponding to different standard deviations from the mean of a normal distribution.

$$Z_T = |T - \mu_T|/\sigma_T.$$

The value we obtain can be compared to the extreme 5% (or other percent) of values of the normal distribution to determine if it is significant or not. The comparison of Z_T can be made more accurate by using a continuity correction, whereby $Z_T = (|T - \mu_T| - \frac{1}{2})/\sigma_T$.

The *Wilcoxon signed-rank test* is similar to the Mann–Whitney test but is used with data that is paired. Paired data describes sets of two values that are linked.

CASE 2.7

Jack has developed a new drug for high cholesterol. He measures the blood cholesterol levels of 10 patients and then administers the drug to each for a period of 3 months. He then measures the patients' cholesterol levels again. His data is presented in Table 2.16.

TABLE 2.16   Effect of Cholesterol Durg After 3 Months

Patient No.	Baseline Cholesterol (mg/dL)	Cholesterol After 3 Months (mg/dL)	Difference Between Baseline and 3-Month Level
1	150	150	0
2	160	170	−10
3	110	90	20
4	155	145	10
5	170	130	40
6	190	210	−20
7	160	160	0
8	180	150	30
9	145	170	−25
10	180	175	5

Assume that the differences are not normally distributed. Is Jack's treatment effective in lowering cholesterol?

In order to use the Wilcoxon signed-rank test, the paired differences must be independent. For example, for patient 3, the fact that the cholesterol decreased by 20 mg/dL neither affects nor is affected by changes in other patients. The first step is to rank all the differences with regard to their magnitude only, i.e., ignoring whether they are positive or negative from smallest to largest. Tied differences are assigned the average rank they would have received had they not been tied. Differences of 0 are simply not ranked and the sample size is reduced by one for each zero difference. Next, we assign the sign of the difference to the ranks and simply add up these ranks. The basic rationale is the following: If the treatment did not have a significant effect, the ranks associated with positive ranks should be similar to those associated with negative ranks, and our total sum should be close to 0.

Table 2.17 includes ranks of magnitudes of differences and their corresponding signs. The sum of ranks is 10. This sum is the *Wilcoxon signed-rank statistic, designated* W. Like the Mann–Whitney test, the magnitude of W is compared to all possible values of rank sums that could occur assuming that the treatment had no effect. For studies with large numbers of pairs,

TABLE 2.17   Ranks of Differences with Corresponding Signs (+/−)

Patient No.	Baseline Cholesterol (mg/dL)	Cholesterol After 3 Months (mg/dL)	Difference Between Baseline and 3-Month Level	Rank of Differences With Sign
1	150	150	0	No rank
2	160	170	−10	−2.5
3	110	90	20	4.5
4	155	145	10	2.5
5	170	130	40	8
6	190	210	−20	−4.5
7	160	160	0	No rank
8	180	150	30	7
9	145	170	−25	−6
10	180	175	5	1

the distribution of W approximates a normal distribution with

$$\mu_W = 0$$

and standard deviation

$$\sigma_W = \sqrt{\frac{n(n+1)(2n+1)}{6}},$$

where n is the number of patients (or pairs of observations).
We can define Z_W as the following test statistic:

$$Z_W = \frac{|W| - 1/2}{\sqrt{n(n+1)(2n+1)/6}}.$$

It is to be compared to the normal distribution. Notice that it includes a *continuity correction*. For Case 2.7, $Z_W = (8 - 1/2)/\sqrt{8\,(8+1)\,(16+1)/6} = 0.54$. Consulting a table of z scores and the corresponding proportion of the normal distribution above and below our value of Z_W reveals that 0.54 is quite close to the mean of the normal distribution and does not represent an extreme value. The cholesterol drug, therefore, did not have a significant effect.

CASE 2.8

Jack now decides to compare his new diet drug to both the old drug and simple nutrition advice to promote weight loss (counseling) among three groups of five patients in a new study. Assume that his observations (Table 2.18) are not normally distributed. Is there a significant difference in effectiveness of the three therapies?

TABLE 2.18 Weight Loss (kg) After 3 Months of Use

New Drug	Old Drug	Counseling
15	4	1
22	3	6
30	4	2
18	4	2
26	9	5

There are more than two groups of non-normally distributed data. To compare these, we use a nonparametric equivalent to ANOVA known as the Kruskal–Wallis test. The procedure begins by assigning a rank to each of the observations regardless of group (lowest rank assigned to smallest observation; tied observations receive average rank of values assuming they were not tied). Next, the rank sum of each group is calculated. The basic rationale is the following: If group assignment has no impact on outcome, the average rank in each group should approximate the average rank of the entire set of observations. Determining how much the average rank in each group deviates from the overall average rank provides a test of this hypothesis.

The overall average rank can be expressed as

$$R_{[\text{overall average}]} = \frac{1+2+3+\cdots+N}{N} = \frac{N+1}{2},$$

where N is the total number of observations.

We can express deviations from this overall average rank by calculating the sum of the squared deviations of each group's mean rank from the overall average rank, and weighting each squared deviation by the number of observations in each group.

$$D = n_1(\overline{R}_1 - R_{[\text{overall average}]})^2 + n_2(\overline{R}_2 - R_{[\text{overall average}]})^2$$
$$+ n_3(\overline{R}_3 - R_{[\text{overall average}]})^2 + \cdots.$$

The Kruskall–Wallis statistic is calculated as

$$H = \frac{D}{N(N+1)/12} \quad \text{or} \quad \frac{12}{N(N+1)} \times \Sigma n_{\text{group}} \left(R_{\text{group}} - R_{[\text{overall average}]}\right)^2.$$

Notice the similarities to ANOVA in how H is calculated.

When there are at least five individuals in each treatment group, the distribution of H approximates the χ^2 distribution with $k-1$ degrees of freedom, where k is the number of groups being compared.

For Case 2.8, the observations with their associated ranks are shown in Table 2.19.

TABLE 2.19   Ranks of Observations by Group

New Drug	Ranks	Old Drug	Rank	Counseling	Rank
15	11	4	6	1	1
22	13	3	4	6	9
30	15	4	6	2	2.5
18	12	4	6	2	2.5
26	14	9	10	5	8

$\overline{R}_{[\text{overall average}]} = 8; \overline{R}_{(\text{new drug})} = 13; \overline{R}_{(\text{old drug})} = 6.4; \overline{R}_{(\text{counseling})} = 4.6.$

$D = 5(13 - 8)^2 + 5(6.4 - 8)^2 + 5(4.6 - 8)^2 = 195.6.$

$H = \dfrac{195.6}{15(15 + 1)/12} = 9.8.$

This value is well above the largest 5% of values of the χ^2 distribution for two degrees of freedom (critical value of 5.991). The three treatments, therefore, are significantly different.

2.13 Correlation

Correlation is a statistical measure of the strength of *association* between two quantitative variables. Association only means that as one variable increases or decreases, the other variable changes proportionately. Correlation does not imply *causation*. For example, the incidence of sunburn may be highly correlated with the number of drownings in a local lake. This does not mean that sunburn causes drowning. The association is likely because both sunburns and drownings occur in hot weather. Case 2.9 illustrates the measurement of correlation.

CASE 2.9

Scientists have been studying the impact of environmental conditions upon pulmonary illnesses for many years. One factor may be hot humid weather. Table 2.20

TABLE 2.20   Temperature and Number of ER Visits for Respiratory Conditions

Day	High Temperature (Washington, DC) (°C)	Number of ER by Adult Visits for Respiratory Conditions
1	29	125
2	25	116
3	32	166
4	31	180
5	35	235
6	36	240
7	33	219
8	39	410
9	35	235
10	29	105

shows the high temperature over a 10-day period in June in Washington, DC, and the corresponding number of records of visits to local emergency rooms (ER) by adults complaining of shortness of breath or worsening emphysema, asthma, or other lung conditions.

Is there an association between temperature and the number of ER visits for respiratory conditions, and if so, how strong is it?

A good way to begin is to plot the data on the chart to visualize a potential association. Such a plot is known as a *scatter diagram* (Fig. 2.6). Since we believe that the number of ER visits depends upon the high temperature, we can describe the temperature as the *independent* variable and the number of ER visits as the *dependent* variable. The independent variable is usually plotted on the horizontal axis. In reality, we are often interested in whether two variables are related and neither one can be described as dependent on the other.

It certainly appears that there is an association between temperature and the number of ER visits. As it gets hotter, the number of ER visits increases. Furthermore, it appears that the relationship between the two variables is *linear*, meaning that the number of ER visits increases proportionately so that we can draw a straight line to approximate the trend.

To describe the strength of the association, we calculate a statistic known as *Pearson's correlation coefficient (r)*. This statistic can assume values between −1 and 1. A value of 1 indicates a perfect positive correlation. That is to say, as one variable increases, the other increases proportionately in a linear fashion. A value of −1 describes a perfect negative correlation. As one variable increases, the other decreases proportionately and linearly.

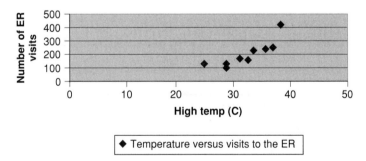

FIGURE 2.6 Temperature Versus Visits to the ER

Pearson's correlation coefficient is calculated as follows:

$$r = \frac{\Sigma(X - \overline{X})(Y - \overline{Y})}{\sqrt{\Sigma(X - \overline{X})^2 \Sigma(Y - \overline{Y})^2}},$$

where X represents the individual values of the independent variable (x or horizontal axis) and Y represents the individual values of the corresponding dependent variable (y or vertical axis). ($\overline{X}$)and ($\overline{Y}$)are the means of the values of X and Y, respectively.

For Case 2.9, ($\overline{X}$) is roughly 32;($\overline{Y}$) is roughly 203. r is quite tedious to calculate by hand. The value of r works out to be 0.90. This means that the correlation between temperature and ER visits is very strong. r^2 is also a very useful quantity. It is a measure of the proportion of variation of the dependent variable that is explained by the independent variable. In Case 2.9, r^2 is 0.81. This can be interpreted in the following way: 81% of the variation in the number of ER visits is accounted for by the high temperature. r^2 is known as the *coefficient of determination*.

We can also determine if the association observed and measured by the correlation coefficient could simply have arisen by chance using a form of the t test given by

$$t = r\sqrt{\frac{(n - 2)}{(1 - r^2)}},$$

where n is the number of pairs of observations. For Case 2.9, $t = 0.9\sqrt{[8 / (1 - 0.81)]} = 5.8$. We now look at our table of t values (see Table A.3) under n–2 degrees of freedom. The critical value of t (two tailed) at a level of significance of 0.05 is 2.306. Since our value exceeds this, it is possible to conclude that the correlation coefficient of 0.9 is statistically significant.

The procedure we just performed to obtain Pearson's correlation coefficient assumes that the two variables being measured are normally distributed. There is a nonparametric equivalent based on ranks known as the *Spearman rank correlation coefficient*.

CASE 2.10

In trying to determine the relationship between the height of palm trees and annual rainfall, you plot the height (m) of a small sample of just 10 trees from different locations in the southern United States and the corresponding annual rainfall (mm) in each location (Table 2.21). Assume that the data are not normally distributed. How strong is the relationship between rainfall and height?

TABLE 2.21   Heights of Trees and Annual Rainfall

Height (m)	Annual Rainfall (mm)
3.5	500
4	720
6	250
5	450
5.5	600
6.5	500
4.5	400
7	550
2	350
9	700

The first step is to determine the difference in ranks (d) for the two variables for each pair of observations. Tied ranks are treated the same way that we discussed with tests of significance. This is shown in Table 2.22.

The Spearman rank correlation coefficient r_S is given by

$$r_s = 1 - \frac{6\Sigma d^2}{n\left(n^2 - 1\right)},$$

where once again n is the number of pairs of observations. For Case 2.9, $r_S = 1 - 6(115.5)/10(100 - 1) = 0.3$. This indicates a weak correlation between rainfall and height. The significance of this correlation is tested in a slightly different way from the Pearson correlation coefficient. A table of critical values of r_S is included in the Appendix (Table A.7). This helps us to determine how significant the trend is between the two variables. At a level of significance of 0.05 and with 10 pairs of observations, the critical value of r_S is 0.648. This means that r_S would have to exceed 0.648 in order to conclude that there is a significant association between rainfall and tree height. When there is no significant association between the two variables, r_S exceeds 0.648 only 5% of the time.

TABLE 2.22 Ranks of Heights and Rainfall, and Differences in Ranks for Each Tree

Height (m)	Annual Rainfall (mm)	Rank of Height	Rank of Rainfall	Difference in Ranks (d)
3.5	500	2	5.5	−3.5
4	720	3	10	−7
6	250	7	1	−6
5	450	5	4	1
5.5	600	6	8	−2
6.5	500	8	5.5	2.5
4.5	400	4	3	1
7	550	9	7	−2
2	350	1	2	−1
9	700	10	9	1

2.14 Regression

Correlation merely describes the strength of association between two variables. The statistical technique of *regression*, by contrast, is much more powerful and is used to assess the precise impact of one or more *predictor* variables upon an outcome variable. For example, we know that a number of factors affect survival of patients with heart failure. These factors include things like a patient's age, class (severity) of heart failure, race, sex, and the presence of other illnesses such as diabetes. These are just three among many possible variables that predict survival time among patients with heart failure. One can describe survival time (the outcome variable) as a *function (f)* of these predictors.

Survival time (days) = f[age (years), class (I, II, III, or IV), race (black, white, Hispanic, Asian, other), sex (male or female), diabetes (yes or no)] + error.

The error term describes the part of the outcome variable of survival time that is not explained by the predictors in the equation. Through regression in theory, we could simply plug in values of age, heart failure class, race, sex, and diabetes status, multiply each by a factor or *regression coefficient* (designated with the symbol β) and obtain an estimate of survival time. The regression coefficient describes the relationship between one predictor variable and the outcome variable. In reality, the situation is more complicated and requires an understanding of statistics that is beyond the scope of this book. Notice that one of the predictor variables (age) is continuous. The remaining are categorical. Class is ordinal; race, sex, and diabetes status are nominal (sex and diabetes status are binary nominal variables). The outcome variable (survival in days) is continuous. *Simple linear regression* involves quantifying the relationship between one continuous predictor variable and one continuous outcome variable when the relationship is best approximated with a straight line. In *logistic regression*, the outcome variable is categorical, usually just two nominal categories, such as disease positive and disease negative. The predictor variables can be of any type. *Ordinal regression*, as you can imagine, deals with outcome variables that are ordinal.

When more than one predictor is used to predict the outcome variable, the technique is known as *multiple regression*. Multiple linear, logistic, and ordinal regression, therefore, involve determining the relationship between more than one predictor variable upon outcomes that are continuous, nominal, and ordinal, respectively.

Of course, the relationship between two continuous variables need not be linear. More advanced statistical techniques are used to quantify relationships in such cases. Physicians are likely to encounter regression in the medical literature as a statistical technique used to quantify relationships between patient or disease characteristics and specific outcomes, such as survival, death, etc. Even the simplest regression equations are usually determined by using statistical computer software rather than by hand. The mathematics can be quite tedious and complicated. For your purposes it is more important to be able to interpret regression analyses accurately. We will next consider two examples of multiple linear regression from published papers with interpretations of the results.

In a recent study, Karnezis and Fragkiadakis wanted to find out what factors determine disability of the wrist in adult patients who had suffered a wrist fracture.[1] The outcome of wrist disability was measured using the patient-rated wrist evaluation score. Patients are asked about pain and their ability to perform certain tasks. A score of zero indicates no wrist disability; 10 is the worst possible score (Table 2.23).

They used multiple regression to determine what factors predicted wrist disability. The most significant factor they found was grip strength:

$$\beta = -1.09, 95\% \, \text{CI} \, (-1.76, -0.42).$$

This should be interpreted in the following way: For every unit of increase in grip strength, the disability score decreases by -1.09, provided other variables remain constant. Notice that the regression coefficient (β) has a 95% confidence interval. Since this interval does not include 0, we can

TABLE 2.23   Patient-Rated Wrist Evaluation Score

Pain (0, no pain; 10, worst ever)
  At rest
  When doing a task with a repeated wrist movement
  When lifting a heavy object
  When it is at its worst
  How often do you have pain? (0, never; 10, always)

Function (0, no difficulty; 10, unable to do)
  Specific activities
    Turn a door knob using my affected hand
    Cut meat using a knife with my affected hand
    Fasten buttons on my shirt
    Use my affected hand to push up from a chair
    Carry a 10-pound object in my affected hand
    Use bathroom tissue with my affected hand
  Usual activities
    Personal care activities (dressing, washing)
    Household work (cleaning, maintenance)
    Work (your job or usual everyday work)
    Recreational activities

conclude that the negative relationship between grip strength and wrist disability is statistically significant.

Lavie, Herer, and Hofstein published a study in the British Medical Journal to determine the relationship between obstructive sleep apnea and blood pressure.[2] Obstructive sleep apnea is a disease characterized by episodes of brief, involuntary, stoppage of breathing at night. The results of their multiple regression analysis among patients not taking drugs for blood pressure are shown in Table 2.24.

According to Table 2.24, for every episode of sleep apnea, the systolic blood pressure rises by about 0.1 and the diastolic blood pressure rises by about 0.07, when other factors are held constant. Age and neck circumference are the two other continuous variables in the *regression model* that have a statistically significant relationship to blood pressure. Sex is a binary, categorical variable. Being male (as opposed to being female) is associated with a decrease in systolic blood pressure of 0.70 (Though not significant statistically, since the 95% confidence interval includes zero. Confidence interval will be discussed later.) and an increase in diastolic blood pressure of 2.05, when other factors are held constant.

TABLE 2.24   Multiple Regression for Factors Affecting Systolic and Diastolic
Pressure

Independent Variables	Systolic Blood Pressure		Diastolic Blood Pressure	
	β (95% CI)	p Value	β (95% CI)	p Value
Apnoea-hypopnoea index (1 apnoeic event)	0.10(0.07–0.13)	0.0001	0.07 (0.05–0.09)	0.0001
Age (1 year)	0.39 (0.34–0.44)	0.0001	0.21 (0.17–0.24)	0.0001
Sex (male)	−0.70 (−2.50–1.11)	0.45	2.05 (0.86–3.24)	0.0007
Neck circumference (1 cm)	1.01 (0.80–1.21)	0.0001	0.47 (0.33–0.61)	0.0001

PROBLEMS

1. The residents of the tiny village of Auckley have suspected for some time that a local chemical plant has been polluting the local water supply. Their general impression is that life expectancy in Auckley is considerably shorter than in other similar communities. A sample of town obituary records reveals the following ages at time of death among 10 adult residents of the town, all of whom passed away in 2007:

   64

   91

   80

   55

   61

   75

   78

   80

   82

   73

   Calculate the mean and standard deviation of age at time of death of the 10 residents.

2. Your friend Jack has just come up with a new treatment for dyslipidemia (high cholesterol) that he calls "Lowerstat." He conducts a

TABLE 2.25   Total Cholesterol Level (mM)

Lowerstat	Strict Diet	Placebo
5.3	6.5	7.0
4.0	6.0	6.8
6.6	5.9	6.5
5.5	7.9	6.6
6.0	8.5	7.8
4.5	5.8	7.7
5.3	5.6	8.0
4.2	6.0	7.8
4.9	7.0	7.7
5.0	6.8	7.3

clinical trial among three groups of 10 patients each to assess the effectiveness of Lowerstat compared to a strict diet and compared to placebo medication. There were no significant differences in cholesterol level among patients in the different groups prior to trial. He measures the cholesterol readings of individual patients after 6 months of therapy. His results are presented in Table 2.25.

Does cholesterol level differ significantly by group?

3. Ignoring the placebo group in Problem 2, is Lowerstat superior to strict diet in lowering cholesterol levels?

4. Two different types of cardiopulmonary resuscitation (CPR) have recently been compared. Standard CPR involves chest compressions alternating with administering breaths; continuous compression CPR (continuous CPR) involves continuous chest compressions only. The impact upon survival is illustrated in the Table 2.26.

TABLE 2.26   Type of CPR and Outcome

Type of CPR	Survived	Died	Total
Standard	20	80	100
Continuous	25	75	100

TABLE 2.27   Depression Scores Before and After 3 Months of Counseling

Patient Number	Initial Depression Score	Score After 3 Months of Counseling
1	12	9
2	18	16
3	15	9
4	13	16
5	17	18
6	8	7
7	5	4
8	10	12
9	14	12
10	15	14

Is continuous CPR superior to standard CPR?

5. The impact of counseling upon depression was recently evaluated in a sample of 10 patients. "Depression scores" are a measure of the severity of depression (20 = extremely depressed; 0 = not depressed at all). Each patient received 3 months of counseling, and the difference in depression scores after 3 months was calculated. The results are shown in Table 2.27. Assume that they are not normally distributed and the change in scores of one patient is independent of any other patient.

Does counseling have a significant impact upon depression scores?

6. Obesity is a risk factor for diabetes. Diabetes is often preceded by elevated fasting levels of the hormone insulin. Table 2.28 shows the data from 10 patients with their body mass index (BMI) (directly proportional to the degree of obesity) and their corresponding fasting insulin level. How strong is the association between BMI and fasting insulin levels? Assume that the data is not normally distributed.

TABLE 2.28 BMI and Fasting Insulin Levels

BMI (kg/m²)	Fasting Insulin Level (IU/mL)
30	65
22	12
36	70
24	8
27	14
40	105
32	50
19	4
21	6
26	16

SOLUTIONS TO PROBLEMS

1. The mean is given by

$$\overline{X} = \frac{\Sigma\,(64 + 91 + 80 + 55 + 61 + 75 + 78 + 80 + 82 + 73)}{10}$$

$$= 74\text{ years.}$$

The standard deviation is given by

$$s = \sqrt{\frac{\Sigma\,\left(X_i - \overline{X}\right)^2}{n-1}}$$

$$= \sqrt{\frac{\Sigma\,\left(X_i - 74\right)^2}{9}}$$

$$= 10.9\text{ years.}$$

2. The correct procedure is ANOVA. The first step is to calculate the grand mean:

$$\text{Grand mean} = \frac{\Sigma x_i}{30}$$

$$= 64.$$

Next, we calculate the total sum of squares:

$$SS_{total} = \Sigma(x_i - \text{grand mean})^2 = \sum(5.3 - 6.4)^2 + (4.0 - 6.4)^2 + \cdots$$
$$= 41.8.$$

The between groups sum of squares is given by

$$SS_{between\ groups} = n\Sigma(\overline{x}_{group} - \text{grandmean})^2$$
$$= 10\Sigma(5.1 - 6.4)^2 + (6.6 - 6.4)^2 + (7.3 - 6.4)^2$$
$$= 25.4.$$

$SS_{within\ groups}$ is therefore $41.8 - 25.4 = 16.4$.

The between groups degrees of freedom is 2. The within number degrees of freedom is $3 \times (10 - 1) = 27$. The between and within groups mean squares are therefore

$$MS_{between\ groups} = 25.4/2 = 12.7.$$
$$MS_{within\ groups} = 16.4/27 = 0.61.$$

F is therefore $12.7/0.61 = 20.8$. The critical value of F at a level of significance of 0.05 is 3.35. Since our value of F greatly exceeds this, there is a statistically significant difference in cholesterol levels among the three groups.

3. The correct statistical test is a t test.

$$t = \frac{\overline{O} - \overline{U}}{\sqrt{s^2/n_{\overline{O}} + s^2/n_{\overline{U}}}}.$$

Our pooled estimate of the variance is given by

$$s^2 = \frac{(n_{\overline{O}} - 1)\,s_{\overline{O}}^2 + (n_{\overline{U}} - 1)\,s_{\overline{U}}^2}{n_{\overline{O}} + n_{\overline{U}} - 2}.$$

The means of the Lowerstat and strict diet groups are 5.1 and 6.6 mM, respectively. The standard deviations of the Lowerstat and strict diet groups are 0.80 and 0.96 mM, respectively.

$$s^2 = \frac{9 \times (0.80)^2 + 9 \times (0.96)^2}{18} = 0.78.$$

$$\text{Therefore, } t = \frac{5.1 - 6.6}{\sqrt{0.78/10 + 0.78/10}} = -3.8.$$

The number of degrees of freedom is $2 \times (10-1) = 18$. The magnitude of the critical value of t at a level of significance of 0.05 (two tailed)

TABLE 2.29 Expected Results Assuming No Difference in Outcomes by Type of CPR

Type of CPR	Survived	Died	Total
Standard	23	77	100
Continuous	23	77	100

is 2.101. Our value exceeds this in magnitude (i.e., absolute value; ignore whether is positive or negative). Lowerstat, therefore, is superior to strict diet.

4. The correct procedure is the χ^2 test.

$\chi^2 = \Sigma\{(|\text{observed–expected value of cell}|-\frac{1}{2})^2/\text{expected value of cell}\}$ (using Yates correction).

Of the 200 patients studied, 45 survived and 155 died. This is a survival rate of 22.5% or roughly 23%. If there had been no difference in survival rates, we would have obtained the values as shown in Table 2.29.

Therefore, χ^2 is (using the Yates correction) $= (|20-23|-\frac{1}{2})^2/23 + (|80-77|-\frac{1}{2})^2/77 + (|25-23|-\frac{1}{2})^2/23 + (|75-77|-\frac{1}{2})^2/77 = 0.48$.

For one degree of freedom, the critical value of χ^2 at a level of significance of 0.05 is 3.84. We can conclude, therefore, that continuous CPR is not superior to standard CPR.

5. These are paired, independent differences. The correct procedure is the Wilcoxon signed-rank test. Table 2.30 shows the differences in scores and their rank with sign.
   The sum of ranks of W is 21.

$$\text{Recall that, } \frac{Z_W = |W|-1/2}{\sqrt{[n(n+1)(2n+1)]/6}} = \frac{21-1/2}{\sqrt{[10(10+1)(20+1)]/6}} = 1.04.$$

We can now compare our value of Z_W to the normal distribution. The proportion of the normal distribution beyond 1.04 standard deviations of the normal distribution on either side of the mean is roughly 15%. A total of 30% of values, therefore, lie either above $Z = 1.04$ or below $Z = -1.04$. The chance of obtaining our results, assuming that that counseling makes no difference, is therefore roughly 30%. This is well above our usual level of significance of 0.05 (5%). We cannot conclude, therefore, that counseling makes a difference.

6. The Spearman rank correlation coefficient is appropriate in this case. Table 2.31 shows the observations with their corresponding ranks and differences in ranks.

TABLE 2.30   Difference in Scores with Signed Ranks

Patient Number	Initial Depression Score	Score After 3 Months of Counseling	Difference	Rank of Difference (With Sign)
1	12	9	3	8.5
2	18	16	2	6
3	15	9	6	10
4	13	16	−3	−8.5
5	17	18	−1	−2.5
6	8	7	1	2.5
7	5	4	1	2.5
8	10	12	−2	−6
9	14	12	2	6
10	15	14	1	2.5

TABLE 2.31   Ranks and Differences in Ranks for Each Patient

BMI (kg/m^2)	Fasting Insulin Level IU/mL	Rank BMI	Rank Insulin	Difference in Ranks
30	65	7	8	−1
22	12	3	4	−1
36	70	9	9	0
24	8	4	3	1
27	14	6	5	1
40	105	10	10	0
32	50	8	7	1
19	4	1	1	0
21	6	2	2	0
26	16	5	6	−1

The Spearman rank correlation coefficient is given by

$$r_s = 1 - \frac{6\Sigma d^2}{n\left(n^2 - 1\right)}.$$

$$d^2 = 1 + 1 + 0 + 1 + 1 + 0 + 1 + 0 + 0 + 1 = 6.$$
$$r_S = 1 - 6 \times 6/[10(10^2 - 1)] = 0.96.$$

This indicates a strong association between BMI and fasting insulin levels.

The critical value of r_S at a level of significance of 0.05 is 0.648. Our value is therefore highly significant.

References

1. Karnezis IA, Fragkiadakis EG. Association between objective clinical variables and patient-related disability of the wrist. *J Bone Joint Surg* 2002;84-B(7):967–970.
2. Lavie P, Herer P, Hoffstein V. Obstructive sleep apnea as a risk factor for hypertension: Population study. *BMJ* 2000;320(7233):479–482.

A Scientific Approach to Diagnosis

3

After reviewing this chapter, you should be able to accomplish the following:

1. Briefly discuss different approaches to diagnosis from a historical perspective.
2. Distinguish between inductive and deductive reasoning.
3. Provide examples of diagnostic reasoning based upon instance-based and prototype-based pattern recognition.
4. Define *screening*.
5. List three essential steps in the evaluation of a new diagnostic test.
6. Define, and given a contingency table, calculate sensitivity, specificity, and positive and negative predictive values.
7. Describe an example of how the prevalence of disease influences positive and negative predictive values.
8. Define *likelihood ratio* (LR).
9. Describe the advantages of using LRs in describing diagnostic tests.
10. Given an appropriate set of data comparing a new diagnostic test to a gold standard, calculate LRs for different types of results.
11. In general terms, describe Bayes theorem and its application to the interpretation of diagnostic test results.
12. Convert odds to probabilities and vice versa.
13. Given the prior odds of disease and the LR for a diagnostic test result, calculate the posterior odds and probability of the disease.
14. Provide an example that illustrates why diagnostic tests are most useful in patients with intermediate pretest probability of disease.
15. List at least three common errors in reasoning that influence the estimation of pretest probabilities of disease.
16. Describe the four phases of diagnostic research.
17. Construct a receiver operator characteristic curve from a small data set to determine the best cutoff of a diagnostic test with dichotomous outcomes.

3.1 Introduction

The word *diagnosis* is derived from the Greek *dia*, meaning *by* and *gnosis*, meaning *knowledge*. Diagnosis is the process of identifying a disease by signs, symptoms, and lab tests as well as the conclusion or conclusions reached through the process—i.e., "Your diagnosis is ...." The process of diagnosis is complex. A good diagnostician certainly needs considerable knowledge of diseases and disease processes. Diagnosticians also need an understanding of different approaches to diagnosis based on different ways of thinking as well as an understanding of quantitative aspects of diagnosis such as determining the probabilities of different diseases. The diagnostic process is characterized by uncertainty, something that many patients do not understand. It is not uncommon to hear things like, "You first told me I had an ulcer and treated me for it. Now you're saying it's something completely different. How can that be?" In addition to medical knowledge, and an understanding of the psychology and quantitative aspects of the diagnostic process, a good diagnostician, therefore, also needs to be able to explain uncertainty in diagnosis to patients in a way they can easily understand. The goal of this chapter is to help you understand how physicians think about diagnosis and how uncertainty in diagnosis can be quantified to make the diagnostic process more rational and transparent to both you and your patients.

3.2 History of Diagnosis

Diagnosis in ancient times was, as you might imagine, by today's standards rather unscientific. Ancient healers and physicians could certainly recognize common diseases and anticipate their consequences. It was hard to mistake small pox or the plague for something else. Ancient diagnosticians, therefore, were skilled observers. They were, however, less concerned with the clinical features of diseases and more with the underlying causes. This became the focus of diagnostic reasoning. In ancient Greece and India, for example, most diseases were thought to be the result of an imbalance of body fluids or *humors*. The Greek physician Hippocrates (after whom the Hippocratic Oath is named) was the first to accurately describe the symptoms and signs of pneumonia. He attributed all disease, however, to an imbalance in the four humors: blood, black bile, yellow bile, and phlegm. Hippocrates believed that it was the imbalance of humors that required diagnosis and treatment. Body fluids served as important diagnostic tools throughout ancient times. Urine was often poured on the ground, for example. A diagnosis of "boils" was made if it attracted insects.

Ancient Greek and Roman medicine, despite its careful attention to observation, was terribly dogmatic. There was no uncertainty. The great Greco-Roman physician Galen combined Hippocrates' four humors with what were then thought to be the four earthly elements (earth, air, fire, and water) to generate diagnoses. Through this diagnostic process, Galen had an explanation for absolutely everything. He was never unsure of any diagnosis. His theories formed the foundation of diagnosis for many centuries thereafter.

In the Middle Ages among Christians in Europe, diagnosis based on humors or anything else became completely unimportant. All diseases were attributed to punishment for sin, spells, or possession by the Devil. It was not until the seventeenth century that diagnosis became more scientific. Englishman William Harvey (1578–1657) discovered the circulation of blood, and mechanical explanations for physiological phenomena soon followed. The first microscope appeared, and physicians and scientists first discovered that microorganisms are the cause of many diseases. Better understanding of anatomy, physiology, and microbiology led to diagnostic techniques designed to detect real pathology. The eighteenth and nineteenth centuries witnessed the development of useful physical examination techniques, such as percussion of the chest, as well as laboratory techniques, such as urinalysis and identification of malaria parasites and the first Roentgenograms (X rays). The Canadian physician William Osler (1849–1919) made huge contributions to the development of modern medicine and, using the rapid developments in clinical and laboratory tools, was among the first to formalize the diagnostic process still used today: A diagnostician begins with a history tailored to the patient, proceeds with an appropriate physical examination, and then obtains laboratory tests if and when they are needed to either confirm suspicions raised by the history and physical examination or rule out certain conditions.

3.3 How Doctors Think About Diagnosis

I have been a practicing physician for more than 10 years, but I still remember how I used to think about diagnosis back in medical school. By the time most medical students begin their clinical rotations, they are skilled information gatherers, also described as *reporters*.[1] This means they are able to accurately and completely gather information from a patient about his current symptoms and history and complete a thorough physical examination keeping in mind any abnormal findings. The student is then able to report this information to a supervising physician in an organized way. After this point, the student is expected to offer his opinion as to the patient's diagnosis. This part is difficult for beginning clinicians. Lack of experience often makes it difficult for the student to come up with any ideas at all about a patient's diagnosis. Gradually, as he accumulates more clinical experience, he gains confidence in offering an idea about diagnosis. Furthermore, his list of potential diagnoses (or *differential diagnosis*) expands to include a number of possibilities often ranked from the most to the least likely. This gradual transformation takes place almost unconsciously. The more clinical experience a student or physician has, the better his diagnostic skill becomes.

There is an extensive body of research about how doctors think about diagnosis—the psychological processes that take place in diagnostic reasoning. At this point, you may wonder about the following question: If physicians become skilled diagnosticians by expanding their knowledge through clinical experience, why is the psychology of diagnostic decision making at all important? There are a couple of important reasons. First, understanding how doctors think about diagnosis raises awareness of one's own diagnostic decision-making processes and the shortcomings associated with such processes. Second, knowledge of the psychology of diagnostic decision making is helpful in designing curricula for learners. The popular problem-based learning movement that is now common in many medical schools in North America, for example, relies heavily upon research into how doctors think about diagnosis.[2]

This section provides an overview of the psychology of diagnostic decision making. This is an evolving field full of controversy. I have included some basic, well-accepted concepts and principles. Consult the bibliography if you wish to know more.

There are many diagnostic strategies used in clinical care. Let us begin with two contrasting, well-established strategies as illustrated in Case 3.1.

CASE 3.1

Arthur is a 24-year-old, third-year medical student beginning his first clinical rotation on an internal medicine ward in a large teaching hospital. One morning he is given two tasks by his supervising physician. For his first task, he is told, "Arthur, I think the patient in room 330 has rheumatic fever. Go find out if he has it or not." For his second task Arthur is told, "The patient in room 405 is feeling unwell and passed out before coming to the hospital this morning. Let me know what you believe she may have." Arthur has very little clinical experience. How do you think he will go about each task? Which task will prove more difficult for him?

Arthur is a clinical novice who may or may not know much about the signs and symptoms of rheumatic fever. Assuming he knows little about it, he will almost certainly open up a textbook (or these days his handheld computer) to a description of rheumatic fever, a condition for which there are specific diagnostic criteria that include such things as arthritis and heart problems. Arthur's task is relatively easy. All he has to do is to check and see if the patient in question meets the diagnostic criteria and provide his supervising physician with a simple "yes" or "no." Of course, if the patient does not meet the diagnostic criteria, Arthur, given his limited clinical experience, would have trouble telling his supervising physician what the patient may actually have. For the second task, Arthur will likely obtain a complete history and conduct a thorough physical examination. Based on this information, he will hopefully come up with a short list of possibilities for the patient's diagnosis. This task is much harder because it requires Arthur not only to gather information but also interpret the information to generate a differential diagnosis.

These two tasks illustrate two basic diagnostic strategies, both of which are used in everyday clinical practice. In the first case, Arthur begins with a particular hypothesis and then tests the hypothesis to see if it is true. He begins by assuming that the patient has rheumatic fever (or assuming he does not) and then determines if the information he gathers is compatible with his initial hypothesis. This is known as *deductive inference* or *deduction* (also known as *hypothetico-deductive* reasoning). In the second case, Arthur does not begin with any hypotheses about diagnosis. He gathers information in order to generate several hypotheses about diagnosis. Most likely, these different hypotheses do not have the same likelihood of being true. This diagnostic reasoning process is known as *inductive reasoning* or *induction*.

Arthur's tasks illustrate two processes that a novice clinician may use. In reality, the processes used in clinical practice, especially by experienced physicians, are more complicated. Whether everyday diagnosis is more likely to be a deductive or inductive process is unclear. Both processes likely play a role in different circumstances. Elstein and Schwarz,[2] based on a review of 30 years of research into diagnostic decision making, identified two distinct philosophies of diagnostic decision making: *problem solving* and *decision making*. This terminology is a little confusing since all diagnosis deals with both problems and decisions. It is possible that one philosophy more than the other accurately describes how doctors think or that both are applicable to clinical practice. Deductive inference is a type of problem-solving strategy. Unlike Arthur, experienced physicians often test more than one hypothesis in a cl_____r. In Arthur's situation, for example, if the patient's prese_____compatible with rheumatic fever, an experienced physicia_____immediately gone on to test the hypothesis of heart failure, _____r some other condition. Deductive inference is not the only_____ng strategy. Quite often, experienced clinicians do not both_____g hypothesis and diagnosis is simply a matter of *pattern recognition* or *categorization*. In other words, for an experienced physician, Arthur's first patient may immediately trigger a pattern (a collection of clinical features) that allows the physician to categorize the patient's diagnosis correctly. The pattern triggered by the patient may be *instance based* or based on a *prototype*. Instance based simply means that the encounter with the patient triggers a memory of a similar patient in the past. This is certainly how many physicians think about skin conditions. A patient with a rash triggers a memory of a patient with a similar pattern that helps establish the diagnosis. In the context of diagnostic decision making, a *prototype* is a typical or ideal pattern constructed in the mind of an experienced physician over time. Years of experience caring for patients with heart failure, for example, helps build a mental prototype which does not exactly fit any specific patient, but is triggered upon encounter with a patient with similar features to the prototype. It is believed that experienced physicians more often rely upon pattern recognition for diagnosis and use deductive reasoning only for especially challenging diagnostic problems.

The second type of diagnostic process, decision making, involves revising opinions about diagnosis based on incomplete or imperfect information. Consider the following example: A man is brought to the emergency room complaining of chest pains. Before seeing the man, you realize that there are a number of different diagnostic possibilities. He could be having a heart attack. He could be having chest pain secondary to a pulmonary or gastrointestinal cause. Perhaps he is anxious and chest pain is a manifestation of his anxiety. Once you enter the room, you realize that he is an elderly man making heart disease more likely. You gather some basic information. It turns out he has been having chest pain for 5 hours. The pain is over the left side of his chest and radiates to his left jaw. He describes it as "crushing" in quality. The man smokes and has high blood pressure and diabetes. Every piece of information causes you to revise what you feel are the chances of the patient having a heart attack. Let us say that before you see him, you consider cardiac, pulmonary, and gastrointestinal causes equally likely (i.e., each has a 33% chance of being correct). As you gather more information, a cardiac cause, such as a heart attack, becomes more likely and the other two categories of causes become less likely. This diagnostic process is illustrated in Fig. 3.1.

In this hypothetical example, each piece of new information raises the chances of a cardiac cause in a stepwise way from 33 to 90%. You do not start with a hypothesis and test it. As you gather information, your list of hypotheses changes. Decision making, in Elstein and Schwarz's terminology, therefore, is an inductive process. The probabilities of different diagnoses at different points in the information-gathering process are quantified using a tool called *Bayes theorem*, which will be explained later in this chapter.

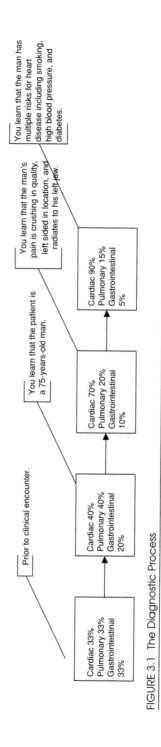

Prior to clinical encounter.

Cardiac 33%
Pulmonary 33%
Gastrointestinal
33%

You learn that the patient is
a 75-years-old man.

Cardiac 40%
Pulmonary 40%
Gastrointestinal
20%

You learn that the man's
pain is crushing in quality,
left sided in location, and
radiates to his left jaw.

Cardiac 70%
Pulmonary 20%
Gastrointestinal
10%

You learn that the man has
multiple risks for heart
disease including smoking,
high blood pressure, and
diabetes.

Cardiac 90%
Pulmonary 15%
Gastrointestinal
5%

FIGURE 3.1 The Diagnostic Process

3.4 Quantifying Diagnosis

The psychology of diagnostic reasoning is interesting and important, but there is some crucial information missing. In Case 3.1, Arthur's suspicion of a cardiac cause of the patient's complaints goes from 33 to 40% as soon as he learns that the patient is a 75-year-old man. Why? Because Arthur knows that the patient's age and sex put him at risk for cardiac disease. Finding out the patient's age and sex can be regarded as a diagnostic test, since it influences the likelihood of different diagnoses. Many people think about diagnostic tests as laboratory tests that include blood or other specimens or radiological tests such as mammograms. Diagnostic tests can be thought of much more broadly. For example, when I evaluate a new patient presenting with a history of frequent headaches, I may begin with one diagnostic hypothesis or several hypotheses. I may wish to know if the patient suffers from migraine. I know that one of the most characteristic features of migraine headache is nausea and vomiting. When I ask the patient, "Do you ever feel nauseated or throw up when you have your headaches?" I am actually performing a diagnostic test with two possible outcomes: yes or no. Similarly, physical examination maneuvers can be thought of us as diagnostic tests. A chest X ray is the best test for pneumonia but physicians also listen to the chest (auscultation) in patients with symptoms suspicious of pneumonia. Auscultation, therefore, can be thought of as a type of diagnostic test for pneumonia. Indeed, diagnosis should be thought of as a series of steps that includes history, physical examination, and laboratory tests each of which leads one closer to a specific diagnosis.

It is time to attach some numbers to diagnostic tests. Diagnostic tests, like the process of diagnosis itself, are subject to uncertainty. This is difficult for many patients to understand who believe that a "positive" test always means they have a particular condition and a "negative" test always means they do not. Explaining the uncertainty associated with test results is among the most challenging tasks in medicine.

CASE 3.2

Colonoscopy is the best way to detect cancer of the colon. Unfortunately, it is expensive and uncomfortable for patients, and not widely available in many parts of the country. Nevertheless, colonoscopy is recommended for all patients aged 50 and over to detect colon cancer whether they have symptoms of the disease or not. The process of identifying disease in people without symptoms is known as *screening*. Your friend Jack has just invented a new test for colon cancer that involves just taking a small blood sample and combining it with a reagent that reacts to cancer cells. Jack developed his test after years of studying the blood of patients with and without colon cancer and identifying certain markers in the blood of patients with cancer that could be identified with a reagent. He asks you to determine the quality of his new diagnostic test. How will you go about this task?

Jack is asking you to evaluate his new diagnostic test. Basically, he wants to know if it correctly identifies patients with colon cancer as having the disease and those without it as not having the disease. The first thing you will need is a group of patients. What kind of patients? You could administer the test to a group of patients known to have colon cancer and see if the test is consistently positive in all of them. If it is positive in all the cancer patients, this may seem impressive. However, what if the test is positive all the time, in both patients with and without colon cancer? Similarly, let us say we "test the test" only in a group of patients known *not* to have colon cancer and the test is negative in all these patients. The test has correctly identified the patients as not having the disease, but perhaps it is negative in many patients who do have the disease as well. This leads us to the first of three important principles in the evaluation of diagnostic tests:

The test should be evaluated among the type of patients who would actually receive the test in clinical practice.

In this case, you would recruit the same types of patients who would normally have colonoscopy, i.e., patients aged 50 and over, in whom it is unknown whether they have cancer or not. It may seem unwise to evaluate the test in patients whose disease status is initially unknown, but their disease status will become clear through a test known as the *gold standard.* The gold standard test for any disease is simply the best test available. It is the test that most closely approximates the truth. Consider a patient whom you suspect to have deep vein thrombosis (blood clot in her leg). There are different tests you can perform. You can examine the leg. You can obtain an ultrasound of the leg. You can also inject a dye into the veins of the leg (venography) to precisely identify a clot. In this case, venography is the gold standard. The gold standard test for colon cancer is colonoscopy. To determine if Jack's test is useful, it should be compared to the gold standard. This is the second important principle in the evaluation of diagnostic tests:

The test should be compared to an appropriate gold standard.

The word *appropriate* is very important. You should not compare Jack's test to some other blood test someone else came up with. The best test is colonoscopy and it should be the only basis for comparison.

Let us say we recruit 100 patients aged over 50 to evaluate Jack's test. In the first patient, Jack's test is negative. In the second patient, Jack's test is positive. We need to compare Jack's test to colonoscopy. Should we

TABLE 3.1   Test Results and Comparison to Disease Findings

	Disease Positive	Disease Negative	Total
Jack's test positive	15	5	20
Jack's test negative	10	70	80
Total	25	75	100

perform colonoscopy in one of the patients and not the other, or both? Suppose we performed colonoscopy in only the patient with a positive test result. We are excluding the possibility that the patient with a negative test result might actually have colon cancer. In other words, we have accepted the negative test result at face value. This makes no sense since the whole idea is to evaluate the quality of Jack's test. Similarly, if we performed colonoscopy only in the patient with a negative test result, we have accepted the positive test at face value. That patient may not have colon cancer. We would not really know unless he had colonoscopy. This leads us to the third important principle:

The gold standard test should be performed in all the patients being studied regardless of the result of the test being evaluated.

In our case, all 100 patients should have both Jack's test *and* colonoscopy. This provides us with a meaningful comparison.

Let us assume that Jack followed this correct methodology. The 2 × 2 contingency table (Table 3.1) shows the results of his test compared to colonoscopy. Since colonoscopy is the gold standard, a positive colonoscopy result can be regarded as definite confirmation of disease or *disease positive.*

Out of 100 patients, 25 have colon cancer. Jack's test identified 15 of them but missed 10. These missed cases are called *false negatives,* since Jack's test incorrectly classified those 10 patients as not having colon cancer. This 15 correctly classified cases are known as *true positives.* Out of these 100 patients, 75 did not have colon cancer. Jack's test correctly classified 70 of them as not having colon cancer, but incorrectly classified 5 of them as having colon cancer. These 5 cases are known as *false positives.* The 70 cases with negative results without cancer are known as *true negatives.* Does Jack's test perform well? Its performance can be quantified with statistics known as *test characteristics.* To define test characteristics not just for Jack's test but for any test and disease with two possible outcomes (usually positive or negative), let us replace Jack's data with algebraic symbols as shown in Table 3.2.

One of the things we would like to know is how many patients with a disease are picked up by a test. This is the *true positive rate,* more

TABLE 3.2   Algebraic Form of Test Results and Disease Status

	Disease +	Disease −	Total
Test +	A	B	A + B
Test −	C	D	C + D
Total	A + C	B + D	A + B + C + D

commonly known as the *sensitivity* of the test. It is simply the ratio of those who test positive and have the disease among all those with the disease, or algebraically

$$\text{Sensitivity} = A/A + C.$$

The higher the sensitivity, the better the ability of a diagnostic test to detect those with disease. Of course, the test may be great at picking up most or all disease, but it is not useful if there are lots of false positives. Another useful test characteristic is the *true negative rate*, better known as the *specificity* of the test. Algebraically

$$\text{Specificity} = D/B + D.$$

The higher the specificity, the better the ability of a diagnostic test to classify patients without the disease correctly.

Jack's test has a sensitivity of $15/15 + 10 = 0.6$ or 60%. It has a specificity of $70/70 + 5 =$ approximately 0.93 or 93%. Its sensitivity can be described as moderate since it only picks up 60% of patients with colon cancer. Its specificity is quite high.

There are two additional test characteristics that are useful in assessing the quality of diagnostic tests with two possible outcomes. In defining sensitivity and specificity, we looked at which patients have or do not have the disease and determined how well the test classified them. We can also look at which patients have positive or negative tests and determine the rates of disease in each group. Consider those who have positive tests; algebraically, this number is $A + B$. Among this group, A is the number who actually have the disease. The rate of true positives over all positives is known as the *positive predictive value* (PPV). Algebraically

$$\text{PPV} = A/A + B.$$

Similarly, among those who have negative tests, the number of true negatives over all negatives is known as the *negative predictive value* (NPV). Algebraically

$$\text{NPV} = D/C + D.$$

With Jack's test, the PPV is $15/15 + 5 = 0.75$ or 75%. The NPV is $70/70 + 10 = 0.88$ or 88%. We would say that according to Jack's data, "75% of those with positive tests actually have colon cancer."

These four test characteristics (sensitivity, specificity, PPV, and NPV) have been confusing generations of medical students, residents, and physicians. Sensitivity is frequently confused with PPV. Specificity is frequently confused with NPV. To clarify, consider the following scenario. Begin by assuming that you have four patients. For the first two patients, you know their disease status and are wondering about the usefulness of a diagnostic test. For the last two patients, you just received their test results and are wondering about their disease status.

Patient 1. To understand the definition of sensitivity, ask yourself:
"I know my patient has the disease. What is the chance that the test will show that my patient has it?" = sensitivity.

Patient 2. For specificity:
"I know my patient does not have the disease. What is the chance that the test will show that my patient does not have it? = specificity.

Patient 3. For PPV:
"I just got a positive test result back on my patient. What is the chance that my patient actually has the disease?" = PPV.

Patient 4. For NPV:
"I just got a negative test result back on my patient. What is the chance that my patient actually does not have the disease?" = NPV.

Remembering this scenario and its four key questions will help you understand the meanings of the four test characteristics and avoid confusion. All these four test characteristics are important in evaluating the usefulness of diagnostic tests. Unlike sensitivity and specificity, which are fixed properties of a test in all circumstances, the PPVs and NPVs of a test change in different circumstances, as illustrated by Case 3.3.

CASE 3.3

The *prevalence* of a disease is simply the proportion of members of a population who have the disease at a particular time (e.g., the prevalence of HIV disease in the United States is roughly 1%). The prevalence of streptococcal pharyngeal infection (strep throat) in a small village of 500 inhabitants is 10%. A new rapid test for detecting strep throat has just been developed. The gold standard test is a throat culture, the result of which takes a couple of days to obtain. It is already known (from a previous study) that the new test has a sensitivity of 90% and a specificity of

95%. The new test is evaluated in all 500 inhabitants and the gold standard (disease positive or negative) is obtained in all of them as well. Construct the corresponding 2 × 2 table and calculate the PPV and NPV. Next, assume that the prevalence of strep throat in another village of 500 people is 20%, rather than 10%, and construct the corresponding 2 × 2 table and calculate the PPV and NPV. In which village is the new test more useful?

Answering the questions raised by the case requires a little arithmetic and logic. In the first village, 10% inhabitants have strep throat. This is 10% of 500 or 50 people. This means that 450 people do not have strep throat. The rapid strep will detect 90% of the 50 cases, or 0.9 times 50 = 45 people. This means it will miss 5 cases. It will correctly classify 95% of those without strep throat or 0.95 times 450 = roughly 428 people. This means it will incorrectly classify 22 as being positive. We now have enough information to construct a 2 × 2 table (Table 3.3).

Algebraically, the PPV is $A/(A + B)$. In this case, PPV = $45/67 = 0.67$ (67%). The NPV is $D/(C + D)$ or $428/433 = 0.99$(99%). This means that if a patient obtains a positive test, there is only a 67% chance that it is a true positive. By contrast, if the patient's result is negative, there is a 99% chance that it is a true negative.

For the second village, the prevalence of 20% means that 20% of 500 or 100 people have strep throat. This means that 400 people do not have strep throat. The rapid strep test will detect 90% or 90 of the 100 cases and therefore miss 10 cases. It will classify 0.95 × 400 or 380 of those without strep throat correctly. This means it will incorrectly classify 20 as being positive. We can construct the 2 × 2 table as shown in Table 3.4.

The PPV is $90/110 = 0.82$ (82%). The NPV is $380/390 = 0.97$(97%). The same test has yielded a significantly higher PPV and a slightly lower NPV. This example illustrates a very important principle of test characteristics:

The sensitivity and specificity are fixed for a given diagnostic test. The PPVs and NPVs, however, vary with the prevalence of disease in the population to which the test is being applied.

TABLE 3.3   Rapid Strep Results in First Village

Rapid Strep Result	Throat Culture Result		
	Disease Positive	Disease Negative	Total
Positive	45	22	67
Negative	5	428	433
Total	50	450	500

TABLE 3.4   Rapid Strep Results in Second Village

| Rapid Strep Result | Throat Culture Result | | |
	Disease Positive	Disease Negative	Total
Positive	90	20	110
Negative	10	380	390
Total	100	400	500

Consider a test with very high sensitivity and specificity. This does not necessarily mean it is always useful in all populations. In a population with a very low prevalence of the disease the test is designed for, the PPV will be low. This means that a relatively high number of the positive test results will be false positives.

CASE 3.4

Your friend Sally has also come up with a new test for colon cancer. Like Jack's test, Sally's test involves obtaining a blood sample and combining it with a reagent. Unlike Jack's test however, Sally's test does not yield two possible outcomes (positive or negative). Much like a weather forecast that predicts high, moderate, or low probability of rain, Sally's test reports high, intermediate, or low probability of colon cancer. Sally performs the test in 1000 people aged over 50. All 1000 then undergo colonoscopy. The results of Sally's test and colonoscopy are compared. The results are shown in Table 3.5. How would you interpret the results?

TABLE 3.5   Test Results and Disease Status

Sally's Test's Result	Disease +	Disease −
High probability	40	10
Intermediate probability	100	150
Low probability	70	630
Total	210	790

Sally's test, unlike Jack's, does not give "*yes*" or *no* (positive or negative) answers about the presence or absence of disease. This means it is not possible to use sensitivity, specificity, and predictive values to determine the quality of the test, since these test characteristics assume two possible outcomes. Tests with two possible outcomes are called *dichotomous*. You might think one way of dealing with this problem is to transform Sally's results into results with two outcomes. For example, we could consider *high probability* and *intermediate probability* as *yes* (positive) and *low probability* as a *no* (negative). Of course, one could argue that instead, intermediate probability should be combined with low probability as a *no* (negative). This is not a correct way to deal with the issue. Sally's test has three types of results for a reason. It is inappropriate to convert these results to something else. We need a new type of statistic or test characteristic.

3.5 Introduction to Likelihood Ratios

The *likelihood ratio* (LR) helps us in situations where a test has more than two possible outcomes. An LR is a ratio of two proportions:

The proportion who have a particular test result (e.g., positive, negative, high probability) among those with a disease *divided by* the proportion who have the same test result among those without the disease.

LRs can be used with any type and number of different test results, whether they include positive, negative, high probability, intermediate probability, low probability, up, down, etc. Algebraically, an LR can be expressed as

$$LR = \frac{\text{Test result/disease} +}{\text{Test result/disease} -}.$$

Let us consider Sally's results and say we wish to calculate the LR for a result of high probability. To calculate the ratio, we begin by determining how often a result of high probability occurs among patients with the disease. In Sally's sample, there are 210 people with the disease, 40 of whom had a result of high probability. How often does a result of high probability occur among people without the disease? There are 790 people without the disease, out of which 10 people have a high-probability result. We now have enough to construct an LR for the result of high probability.

$$LR \left(\text{high probability}\right) = \frac{40/210}{10/790} = 15.$$

We would interpret this LR in the following way: "A result of high probability is 15 times more likely to occur among people with colon cancer than among people without colon cancer." This may seem like a convoluted way of saying that a result of high probability means that a patient has a high chance of having cancer. Although the meanings of LRs are not intuitively obvious to most physicians, their usefulness will become apparent in Section 3.7.

As we did for high probability, we can also calculate the LRs for Sally's intermediate- and low-probability results.

$$\text{LR (intermediate probability)} = \frac{100/210}{150/790} = 2.5,$$

$$\text{LR (low probability)} = \frac{70/210}{630/790} = 0.41.$$

According to this data, does a high-probability result mean that a patient has the disease? Does a low-probability result rule disease out? How about an intermediate-probability result? In general, a result with an LR over 10 makes the presence of disease very likely. If Sally's test was performed on a patient and the result was "high probability," this would make it very likely that the patient had colon cancer. LRs of 0.1 or nearly as small mean that disease is very unlikely and effectively ruled out. Unfortunately, a result of low probability with Sally's test, therefore, does not rule out disease. A result with a LR 1.0 is not at all useful in ruling in or ruling out disease. We will more precisely quantify the relationships between LRs and their impact on the likelihood of disease in Section 3.7.

3.6 LRs and Sensitivity and Specificity

As mentioned before, LRs can be used with tests that have any number of different outcomes. With tests with dichotomous outcomes, LRs have a simple algebraic relationship to sensitivity and specificity. Let us return to our algebraic 2 × 2 contingency table (Table 3.6).

There are only two possible test results (+,–). Let us calculate the LR for a + test. A + C people have the disease. A positive test occurs "A" times among them. B + D people do not have the disease. A positive test occurs "B" times among them. Our LR is therefore

$$LR(+) = \frac{A/(A+C)}{B/(B+D)}.$$

The numerator of this LR should seem familiar. $A/(A + C)$ is the sensitivity of the test. Recall that $D/(B + D)$ is the specificity. Since $D/(B + D) + B/(B + D) = 1$, therefore $B/(B + D) = 1 - D/(B + D)$. The

TABLE 3.6   Algebraic 2 × 2 Table

	Disease +	Disease –	Total
Test +	A	B	A + B
Test –	C	D	C + D
Total	A + C	B + D	A + B + C + D

denominator is therefore, 1 – specificity. The LR of a positive test (positive LR) can therefore be expressed as

$$LR(+) = \frac{\text{sensitivity}}{1 - \text{specificity}}.$$

The LR of a negative test result can be expressed algebraically as

$$LR(-) = \frac{C/(A + C)}{D/(B + D)}.$$

The denominator is the specificity of the test. The numerator is 1 – sensitivity. The LR of a negative test (negative LR) is therefore

$$LR(-) = \frac{1 - \text{sensitivity}}{\text{specificity}}.$$

Given the sensitivity and specificity of a test, the positive and negative LRs can therefore be calculated easily.

3.7 LRs and Bayes Theorem

Thomas Bayes (1702–1761) was an English mathematician and Minister whose simple theorem that describes how new information should be used has found many applications in the design of medical research studies and in medical decision making. The significance of Bayes' work was not recognized until after his death. His friend Richard Price discovered a paper Bayes wrote, called an *Essay towards solving a problem in the doctrine of chances,* and sent it for publication to the *Philosophical Transactions of the Royal Society of London* in 1764. In an introduction to the essay, Price wrote,

> *I now send you an essay which I have found among the papers of our deceased friend Mr Bayes, and which, in my opinion, has great merit... In an introduction which he has writ to this Essay, he says, that his design at first in thinking on the subject of it was, to find out a method by which we might judge concerning the probability that an event has to happen, in given circumstances, upon supposition that we know nothing concerning it but that, under the same circumstances, it has happened a certain number of times, and failed a certain other number of times.*[3]

Essentially, *Bayes theorem* states that in determining the probability that an event will happen, we should take into consideration the circumstances under which it has happened in the past. It is a mathematical rule explaining how existing opinions (prior beliefs) should be changed in light of new evidence. This may seem uncontroversial but applications of Bayes theorem, particularly to the design and interpretation of clinical trials can be very complex and are the subject of considerable debate. A major source of controversy is the legitimacy of quantifying prior beliefs. An elegant imaginary example of how this can be done is the following[4]: Imagine a newborn who witnesses his first sunrise. He wonders if he will observe the phenomenon again and assigns equal probability to a sunrise the next day or no sunrise the next day and places a white ball and a black ball in a bag (i.e., 50% chance of the sun rising again). The next day, the sun rises again. He places another white ball in the bag. In his scheme, based on his prior beliefs, the sun now has a two-third chance of occurring again. As the sun rises each day, he places another white ball in the bag. In a very short time, the rising of the sun becomes a near certainty based on his prior beliefs. Each new sunrise is interpreted in conjunction with prior belief to draw conclusions about what will happen in the future. A very general form of Bayes theorem can be expressed as

$$\text{Prior odds of hypothesis} \times \text{Bayes Factor} = \text{Final (posterior) odds of hypothesis.}$$

Odds will be explained in the next section. *Prior odds* simply represents the strength of prior belief. In the aforementioned example, it is the ratio of white to black balls. The Bayes factor represents new information (in whatever form). In this example, the new information is each additional sunrise. As applied to diagnostic tests, Bayes theorem can be expressed as

$$\text{Pretest odds of disease} \times \text{LR} = \text{Posttest odds of disease.}$$

We have already, therefore, discussed one tool for the use of Bayes theorem for diagnostic test results. The LR represents the Bayes factor or new information. The LR of the test result is multiplied by the pretest odds to obtain the posttest odds of disease.

3.8 Odds and Probabilities

Bayes theorem for diagnostic tests makes use of odds instead of probability because it allows us to use the aforementioned equation, which takes the form of a simple linear relationship. Probability is simply a measure of how likely it is that an event will occur. Most people have a good understanding of the meaning of probability. When a weather forecast indicates that there is a 40% probability of rain, we understand that there is a 4 in 10 chance of rain and a 6 in 10 chance of no rain. Odds are not as intuitively obvious to physicians or others. Physicians use probabilities all the time. For example, "There is a 50% probability of survival after one year." Those familiar with betting on horses and other games of chance, however, are familiar with odds. When a horse is described as a 30:1 longshot of winning, this means the horse has one chance of winning and 30 chances of losing. Odds are the frequency of one event occurring versus another and can be easily obtained from a probability. Let us say the probability of a patient having lung cancer is 33% (or 0.33 or one-third). What are the corresponding odds? The patient has a 33% chance of having lung cancer and therefore has a 67% (0.67) chance of not having lung cancer. The odds is simply the ratio of

$$\frac{\text{Probability of having disease}}{\text{Probability of not having disease}} = 33\%/67\%$$

$$= \frac{1}{2} \, (\text{or 1 in favor to 2 against}).$$

Since patients either have or do not have a disease, the probability of not having a disease can be expressed as 1 – the probability of having disease (or 100 – probability of having disease, if probability is expressed in percent terms). The relationship of odds to probability can be more generally expressed as

$$\text{Odds} = \text{probability}/(1 - \text{probability}).$$

If the probability of disease is 0.5, the corresponding odds are $0.5/1 - 0.5 = 1/1$, or 1 in favor to 1 against. We can also convert from odds to probability. Let us say that the odds of disease are expressed as 1 to 2 (1/2). The probability of disease is given by

$$\text{Probability}(p) = \frac{\text{odds in favor}}{\text{odds in favor} + \text{odds against}}.$$

The odds in favor + odds against is a sum also known as the total odds. In our example,

$$p = 1/1 + 2 = 0.33 \, (\text{or 33\%}).$$

3.9 Applying Bayes Theorem

We now have the tools we need to use Bayes theorem with diagnostic tests. As an example, consider a patient who wants to know if she has colon cancer, but does not want a colonoscopy. She requests Sally's test from her doctor. To apply Bayes theorem, we need a measure of pretest probability (or odds). This is the probability that the patient has colon cancer before the test result is obtained. The patient feels generally well but has a strong family history of colon cancer. Let us say our subjective impression is that the patient has a pretest probability of colon cancer of 5%. Her odds of colon cancer are therefore given by

$$\text{Odds} = p/1 - p = 0.05/1 - 0.05 = 1/19.$$

Her odds of having cancer versus not having cancer are 1 to 19. Now let us say the doctor performs the test and the result returns as *high probability*.

What does this mean? We know that this result has an LR of 15. We can now calculate the posttest odds of disease as

$$\text{Posttest odds} = 1/19 \times 15 = 15/19.$$

This translates to a posttest probability of

$$15/15 + 19 = 0.44(44\%).$$

Using Bayes theorem and obtaining a test result of high probability, the patient's probability of colon cancer has gone from 5 to 44%. This is quite a high probability of colon cancer. Colonoscopy is the gold standard for diagnosis. Informing the patient that, based on Sally's test, she has a 44% chance of having colon cancer might persuade her to have a colonoscopy. This is the way in which many diagnostic tests are used in clinical practice. An initial test is provided to a large population that is at risk for a disease but has no symptoms. Those who test positive then receive a confirmatory test (gold standard). Sally's test, therefore, can be used as a screening test to determine who should have colonoscopy.

One aspect of this chapter may now strike you as particularly *unscientific*. I told you our subjective impression of the patient's probability of having colon cancer is 5%. The classic imaginary example of Bayes theorem whereby a baby adds a white ball to a bag with every witnessed sunrise provides a way to precisely quantify the pretest or prior probability of an event. In reality, the pretest odds used with diagnostic tests are a subjective impression based upon clinical experience or clinical experience combined with data from similar patients. This is a source of controversy in the application of Bayes theorem. It is important to keep in mind that medical decision making often involves combining subjective impressions with scientific data. This does not make Bayes theorem unscientific. Case 3.5 illustrates the influence of Bayes theorem upon three different patients.

CASE 3.5

A new test for myocardial infarction (*heart attacks*) is being used in an emergency department. It provides a result in just a couple of minutes, compared with several hours for the gold standard test. Prompt treatment of myocardial infarction is necessary to prevent permanent heart damage or death. Unfortunately, the treatment itself carries significant risks. The test has a positive LR of 5 and a negative LR of 0.2. Descriptions of three different patients who present with chest pain are given next. First, assume that for each patient, the test is positive. Next, assume that the test is negative. How did the test result influence medical decisions in each case? In which patient is the test most useful?

> *Patient 1*: Mr. D. is an obese 60-year-old smoker with a long-standing history of diabetes, high blood pressure, and high cholesterol who complains of 2 hours of "crushing" retrosternal chest pain.
>
> *Patient 2*: Ms. A is a 21-year-old college student who complains of episodic "twinges" in the left side of her chest for the past 2 days. She does not smoke, take any medications, or have any medical history of significance. She admits to being under a great deal of stress recently as final exams are about to begin.
>
> *Patient 3*: Mr. Y is a 47-year-old smoker who complains of an "unusual pressure" in his chest for the past 5 hours. He has not had symptoms of this type before. He has no history of hypertension, diabetes, dyslipidemia, or family history of heart disease. He exercises regularly without any chest discomfort.

It does take some clinical experience to make a reasonable guess as to each patient's chances of having a heart attack. The first patient has many risk factors for heart disease including obesity, smoking, diabetes, high blood pressure, and high cholesterol. He also has pain that is typical of someone having a heart attack. Without any testing at all, a reasonable guess of his chances of having a heart attack is 75%. By contrast, Ms. A has no risk factors for heart disease. Heart attacks are virtually unheard of in patients her age. The information provided suggests that anxiety or stress may be the cause of her "twinges." Let us estimate her chances of having a heart attack as 1%. Finally, Mr. Y is a smoker. His description of "unusual pressure" is somewhat vague. He is neither particularly young nor especially old. He presents a diagnostic challenge. Let us estimate his chances of having a heart attack as 25%. Now let us first determine how a negative test influences these pretest probabilities. We need to convert each of the pretest probabilities to odds and multiply by the negative LR of 0.2 to obtain posttest odds. As described before, these can be easily converted back to probabilities. Table 3.7 provides a summary of the three patients.

Now let us assume the heart attack is positive. The pretest odds are multiplied by 5 (Table 3.8).

TABLE 3.7   Test for Heart Attacks is Negative

	Pretest Probability (%)	Pretest Odds	Posttest Odds	Posttest Probability
Mr. D	75	3/1	0.6/1	0.38 (38%)
Ms. A	1	1/99	0.0002/1	0.0002 (0.2%)
Mr. Y	25	1/3	0.067/1	0.063 (6.3%)

TABLE 3.8   Test for Heart Attacks is Positive

	Pretest Probability (%)	Pretest Odds	Posttest Odds	Posttest Probability
Mr. D	75	3/1	15/1	0.94 (94%)
Ms. A	1	1/99	5/99	0.048(4.8%)
Mr. Y	25	1/3	1.67/1	0.62 (62%)

Let us consider how the two possible test results influenced decision making in each case. Mr. D, prior to the test, already had a 75% chance of having a heart attack. Even with a negative test, his chances remain a substantial 38%. Most physicians would be wary about attributing his chest pain to something other than a heart attack given a 38% probability of a heart attack. Such a patient would likely remain in hospital under careful observation, or even treated for a heart attack pending the results of a gold standard test. With a positive test, Mr. D's chances increase from 75 to 94%. This makes a heart attack even more likely, but it is unlikely that a physician would treat a patient differently with a 94% probability versus a 75% probability. With a positive test or with no test result available at all, Mr. D would likely remain in hospital and receive prompt treatment.

With a negative test, Ms. A's chances of having a heart attack decline from 1 to 0.2%. With a positive test, her chances increase to 4.8%. In either case, the test is unlikely to influence management. Even with a positive test, Ms. A would not receive treatment for a heart attack. Her physician would likely look for other causes of her pain, and her evaluation could take place in an outpatient clinic rather than the hospital.

With a negative test, Mr. Y's chances of having a heart attack decline from 25 to 6.3%; with a positive test, the chances increase to a substantial 62%. If no test was available and he presents with a 25% chance of a heart attack, he would most likely be admitted to hospital for observation. He may or may not receive treatment. With a 62% chance, he would certainly be admitted and most likely receive prompt treatment. With a 6.3% chance, another cause of his pain would be considered and admission to hospital would likely be considered unnecessary. It is easy to see that in his case, the test has the most influence on medical decision making. Decisions do not change significantly with either type of test result in the cases of Mr. D and Ms. A. This case illustrates a very important principle:

Diagnostic tests are most useful in patients with intermediate pretest probabilities of disease.

Intermediate pretest probability is a somewhat vague term. It can be defined as a probability or range of probability at or within which decisions about diagnosis or patient care are uncertain.

3.10 Errors in the Estimation of Pretest Probabilities

As mentioned, the pretest or prior probabilities used in Bayes theorem are subjective. They are based on clinical experience and could be described as "hunches" about the likelihood of disease. Use of Bayes theorem is controversial partly because estimation of pretest probability is prone to certain common errors in thinking that have been extensively studied. This section includes a description of some of the most common errors.

Cases of the severe acute respiratory syndrome (SARS) virus began appearing in Toronto in early 2003. The virus causes severe respiratory disease, and a number of deaths had been reported in the Far East. Symptoms of SARS infection at first resemble any flu-like illness. SARS received an enormous amount of media attention across Canada and the United States. Despite the fact that influenza and the "common cold" are far, far more common than SARS, during the spring of 2003, many physicians became concerned that their patients with flu-like symptoms had SARS. Before obtaining any tests for SARS, physicians were likely to overestimate the pretest probability of SARS simply due to the attention the disease was receiving in the media, medical community, and general public. This is an error based on *availability* of memories or information. People tend to overestimate the frequency of vivid events (e.g., SARS infections) and underestimate the frequency of ordinary events (e.g., common cold).

People overestimate the probability of disease based on how similar or *representive* a case is to a prototype. Consider the following example: A young man who works for a specialized company that removes asbestos from old buildings presents with cough, wheezing, and occasional shortness of breath. These symptoms are characteristic of asbestosis but also the far, far more common disease of asthma. Prior to any testing, his probability of having asbestosis is likely to be overestimated and probability of having asthma underestimated because his symptoms together with a history of working with asbestos fit the prototype of asbestosis, even though asthma is more common. Overestimation based on the representiveness of a case to a prototype is related to a phenomenon known as the *conjunction fallacy*. This is the incorrect conclusion that the probability of a joint event is greater than the probability of any one of the events alone. The classic example of the conjunction fallacy was described by Nobel prize winners Tversky and Kahneman.[5]

Linda is 31 years old, single, outspoken, and very bright. She majored in philosophy. As a student, she was deeply concerned with issues of discrimination and social justice, and also participated in antinuclear demonstrations.

Which is more likely?

1. Linda is a bank teller.

2. Linda is a bank teller and is active in the feminist movement.

Eighty-five percent of the people presented with this problem selected choice 2, which is incorrect. Linda may fit the prototype of someone active in the feminist movement, but the joint probability of her being both a bank teller and active in the feminist movement must be less than probability of her being a bank teller. In the diagnostic process, we may at first encounter a patient who presents with several characteristics that are 'stereotypical' of a disease (e.g. an elderly man with weight loss *and* anemia *and* history of smoking, in whom we suspect colon cancer). The conjunction fallacy only tells us to formulate our pre-test probability cautiously, since in any given patient, a combination of findings is less likely to occur than any single finding alone.

There are several other ways through which pretest probability is prone to error. *Support theory* claims that an estimate of the probability of an event depends upon how detailed is its description. A patient who provides a careful, detailed description of symptoms characteristic of a heart attack, for example, may elicit a higher pretest probability of disease than a patient who gives a more succinct description, even if both descriptions contain exactly the same information related specifically to heart attacks. Another common error is the *overemphasis of positive findings and under emphasis of negative findings* in conducting a clinical evaluation. This can lead to overestimation of pretest probability. The Annotated Bibliography includes a list of references where you can learn more about these and other errors in estimation of probability.

3.11 Diagnostic Research

Case 3.2 describes the basic methodology of determining the usefulness of a diagnostic test: An appropriate group of patients is assembled; all patients receive the diagnostic test and a suitable gold standard; the diagnostic test results are compared to the gold standard results to determine test characteristics. This type of evaluation—though the most likely you will encounter in the medical literature and arguably the most important—is just one type of research in the development of diagnostic tests. Sackett and Haynes define four types of questions or phases of diagnostic research.[6] Let us say that we wish to develop a new type of test for lung cancer and have identified a new blood marker, called Q, that someone noticed seems to be elevated in patients with lung cancer. The first phase of diagnostic research (*Phase I*) is to determine if the levels of Q differ significantly between patients with and without the disease. In Phase I, therefore, we are not carrying out the test in patients who are at risk for the disease or would normally get the test in clinical practice. We are simply trying to determine if the test has the potential to distinguish people with and without the disease. Let us say, in comparing levels of Q among 100 patients known not

Levels of Q

	Patients With Lung Cancer	Patients Without Lung Cancer
Mean level of Q (μg/dL of blood)	36.5	14.8

to have lung cancer and 100 patients known to have lung cancer, we find the following data:

The mean level of Q is much higher in patients with cancer. In *Phase II*, we ask, "Are patients with certain test results more likely to have the disease than patients with other test results?" In this phase, we start by obtaining levels of Q and then finding out which levels of Q are associated with disease. In Phase I, we went in the opposite direction. We started by knowing who had cancer and who did not and obtained levels of Q. In Phase II, for example, we may notice that almost all patients with levels of Q higher than 20 μg/dL had lung cancer, while almost all patients with levels of Q less than 10 μg/dL did not. It is in this phase that we often obtain *cutoffs* for different types of test results. This process is illustrated in Case 3.6.

CASE 3.6

A new "questionnaire" test has been developed to determine if a patient is suffering from a migraine headache. The patient simply answers the questions given in Table 3.9. One point is assigned to each *yes*.

TABLE 3.9   Migraine Diagnostic Questionnaire

1.	Are you female?	Yes	No
2.	Is your headache on one side of your head only?	Yes	No
3.	Would you describe your headache as throbbing?	Yes	No
4.	Do you feel nauseated?	Yes	No
5.	Does exertion (e.g., running, lifting heavy objects) make your headache worse or bring on headaches in general?	Yes	No
6.	Do bright lights aggravate your headache?	Yes	No
7.	Do loud sounds aggravate your headache?	Yes	No
8.	Do you have a family history of migraines?	Yes	No

The questionnaire was administered to 200 headache sufferers. All 200 were then evaluated by a headache specialist who decided whether the patient had a migraine or not through a detailed interview (i.e., the headache specialist's evaluation was the gold standard). The number of positive responses among different

headache sufferers was compared to the specialist's diagnosis of migraine. The
results are given in Table 3.10.

TABLE 3.10   Number of Responses and Disease Status

Number of *Yes* Responses	Positive Diagnosis of Migraine (+)	No Diagnosis of Migraine (−)
0	0	16
1	2	34
2	2	16
3	16	20
4	16	8
5	20	4
6	24	2
7	10	0
8	10	0

How would you use this information to develop an appropriate cutoff for the new
headache questionnaire?

To simplify things, let us say we wish to use the headache questionnaire to
develop a test with dichotomous (positive or negative) outcomes. We can
then use the familiar test characteristics of sensitivity and specificity. We
could use a certain number of positive responses as a cutoff between positive migraine and negative migraine. What should the cutoff be? Let us say
we believe that two or more positive responses should constitute an appropriate cutoff. Out of 100 people with migraine headaches, 98 have two or
more positive responses. Unfortunately, 50 out of 100 people without migraine headaches also have two or more responses. Let us now construct
a 2 × 2 table using two or more responses as a cutoff (Table 3.11).

TABLE 3.11   2 or more Responses

Number of + Responses	Migraine +	Migraine −
≥2 (i.e., positive)	98	50
<2 (i.e., negative)	2	50
Total	100	100

We can now calculate the sensitivity and specificity of the question-naire using this cutoff. The sensitivity is 98/98 + 2 = 98%. This is a very good sensitivity. Unfortunately, the specificity is only 50/50 + 50 = 50%. With a cutoff of 2, therefore, the test is highly sensitive and detects most migraines. It also has, however, an unacceptably large number of false positives (poor specificity).

Let us consider three other cutoffs: cutoffs of seven or more positive responses, three or more positive responses, and four or more positive responses. The corresponding 2 × 2 contingency tables (Tables 3.12–3.14) are shown next.

TABLE 3.12   Seven or More Positive Responses

Number of + Responses	Migraine +	Migraine −
≥7 (i.e., positive)	20	0
<7 (i.e., negative)	80	100
Total	100	100

In this case, the sensitivity is just 20% and the specificity is 100%.

TABLE 3.13   Three or More Positive Responses

Number of + Responses	Migraine +	Migraine −
≥3 (i.e., positive)	96	34
<3 (i.e., negative)	4	66
Total	100	100

The sensitivity is 96% and the specificity is 66%.

TABLE 3.14   Four or More Positive Responses

Number of + Responses	Migraine +	Migraine −
≥4 (i.e., positive)	80	14
<4 (i.e., negative)	20	86
Total	100	100

The sensitivity is 80% and the specificity is 86%.

Among these four cutoffs, clearly four or more positive responses is the only one with reasonably high sensitivity and high specificity. Determining the optimal cutoff for a diagnostic test with two outcomes is always a tradeoff between sensitivity and specificity. We could continue constructing 2 × 2 tables for all possible cutoffs. The optimal cutoff can be determined using what is known as a receiver operator characteristic (ROC) curve. The name comes from aviation. ROC curves were developed to analyze the quality of radar. An ROC is a plot of sensitivity against 1–specificity.

The goal in deciding upon a cutoff is to optimize both sensitivity and specificity. In other words, we want to maximize the number of true positives and minimize the number of false positives. An ROC curve is constructed by plotting the sensitivity against 1–specificity for different cutoffs. The optimal cutoff is the one that is closest to the upper left-hand corner of the graph. In Fig. 3.2, for example, the optimal cutoff is 7. ROC curves can also be used to compare different diagnostic tests. The area under an ROC curve is a measure of its discriminant ability—its ability to distinguish between those with and without disease. Since sensitivity and 1 – specificity can both be expressed as a number from 0 to 1, the maximum possible area under an ROC curve is a square with an area of 1.

Three different tests are represented in Fig. 3.3. The area under the dashed curve is greatest. It is therefore the best diagnostic test overall. The test represented by the solid curve is next best. The test represented by the dotted-line curve is completely useless in distinguishing between those with and without disease. The area under it is 0.5.

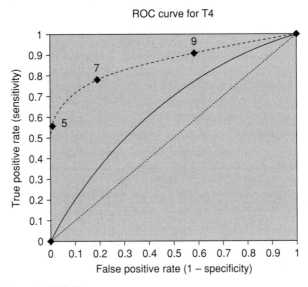

FIGURE 3.2 Sample ROC Curve

Comparing ROC curves

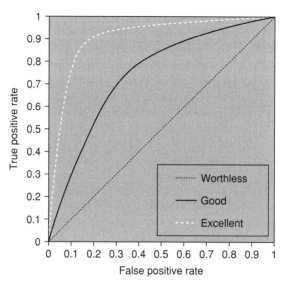

FIGURE 3.3 Comparing ROC Curve

ROC curves have another interesting property. Recall that with a test with dichotomous outcomes, the positive LR is given by sensitivity/(1 – specificity). Sensitivity and 1 – specificity are what is plotted on an ROC curve. The slope of a tangent to an ROC curve at any given point is the ratio sensitivity/(1 – specificity), i.e., the LR. The curve designated "worthless" in Fig. 3.3 is a straight line with the same slope of 1.0 at all points. The corresponding LR is therefore 1.0. From Bayes theorem we know that an LR of 1.0 does not change pretest odds at all. A test result with an LR of 1.0 is completely useless in medical decision making.

Phase III diagnostic research is the familiar research described in Case 3.2. A new test is evaluated in a group of patients likely to have the test in clinical practice and the results are compared to a suitable gold standard to determine test characteristics. In *Phase IV*, diagnostic research, we ask the question, do patients who have a diagnostic test fare better than those who do not? For example, let us say that Jack's test for colon cancer has been around for several years. Presumably the test allows us to detect more colon cancer, treat it sooner, and allow more patients to survive. This may not be true for several reasons. Perhaps the test allows us to pick up disease earlier, for example, but earlier treatment makes no difference to long-term survival. To address these types of questions, we could compare patients who have and do not have the test over a period of time to see if having the test improves outcomes. In this sense, the diagnostic test is actually a type of therapy. The evaluation of therapies will be discussed in Chapter 4.

PROBLEMS

1. A new quick blood test ("Quick Test") for myocardial infarction (*heart attack*) was recently evaluated in a group of 1000 patients with acute on-set of chest pain. Results are reported as "highly likely," "likely," "pos-sible," and "unlikely." All 1000 patients subsequently underwent for-mal serum enzyme testing (gold standard) to identify those with and without myocardial infarction. The results of both tests were then com-pared, as shown in Table 3.15.

   Calculate the LRs for all four types of Quick Test results based on the aforementioned data.

2. The manufacturer of the Quick Test decided to simplify the way in which results are reported. Now, results that were originally reported as highly likely or likely are simply considered "positive," those that were originally reported as "possible" or "unlikely" are now reported simply as "negative." Using the same data in Problem 1, construct a 2 × 2 table for positive and negative Quick Test results. Calculate the sensitivity, specificity, PPV and NPV for the Quick Test.

3. You are suspicious that a patient in your office has pneumonia. The pa-tient is a young woman with a fever of 39°C and productive cough. You estimate that her probability of having pneumonia upon presentation is 75%. Her health insurance does not cover the cost of medications, and she does not want to take antibiotics if it can be avoided at all. She is extremely fearful that something more sinister than pneumonia is going on and insists that you obtain a chest X ray. The chest X ray, when interpreted by a skilled physician like you, has a positive LR of 4 and negative LR of 0.6 for pneumonia.

TABLE 3.15   Quick Test Results and Disease Status

Quick Test Result	Confirmatory Test +	Confirmatory Test −
Highly Likely	80	20
Likely	120	80
Possible	240	300
Unlikely	4	156

The patient's chest X ray is completely normal (i.e., negative).

What is her posttest probability of pneumonia? If she had not been so insistent about an X ray, would you have obtained one given the information here? Why or why not?

4. You come across a new paper describing a new diagnostic test for Parkinson disease. The diagnostic test uses a new device known as a "Manual Oscillometer" that measures tremor frequency and amplitude and calculates the probability of Parkinson disease. The investigators evaluated the new device on 120 hospital employees aged 18–68. Eighteen people tested positive on the oscillometer test. All 18 were contacted by telephone and given their results. They were asked to see a neurologist of their choice within 1 month. The 18 patients saw 4 different neurologists. The charts of the patients from the neurologists' office were reviewed 6 months later to see which of the patients had been diagnosed with Parkinson disease. Among the 18 positive test results, 16 of the patients were diagnosed with Parkinson disease (PPV = 16/18 = 89%). The investigators describe this result in their paper as "very impressive." What is wrong with the investigators' methodology?

5. A 60-year-old man with a history of smoking, high blood pressure, and diabetes presents to an emergency room complaining of vague abdominal and chest pain. Which of the two possibilities given next has the highest probability?

   a. The man gets very little exercise.

   b. The man gets very little exercise and is suffering from a heart attack.

6. Cystic fibrosis (CF) is a serious inherited disorder that occurs in about 1/2500 live births. Identifying CF is cumbersome and requires either genetic testing, which is not available in many areas, or testing of sweat chloride, which is difficult and often inaccurate. Your friend Jack believes that blood levels of the newly identified enzyme lipase-beta can be used to diagnose CF. He measured lipase-beta levels in 100 newborns born to couples in which either the mother or father or both carry the CF gene. He then performed genetic testing on all 100 of these babies to determine the accuracy of his test. Lipase-beta is measured in increments of 10 μg/dL only. Levels below 10 μg/dL cannot be measured accurately. Your task is to determine the best lipase-beta "cutoff" score for a positive test. Jack's data are given in Table 3.16.

TABLE 3.16   Lipase β Level and Disease Status

Level of Lipase-beta (μg/dL)	CF+ by Genetic Testing	CF− by Genetic Testing
10	1	32
20	2	24
30	8	11
40	8	3
50	10	1

SOLUTIONS TO PROBLEMS

1. Recall that an LR is the ratio of how often a test result occurs among people with a disease over how often it occurs in people without a disease. There are 444 people with the disease and 556 without disease. The LRs are therefore the following:

   LR(highly likely) = 80/444/20/556 = 0.18/0.036 = 5

   LR(likely) = 120/444/80/556 = 0.27/0.14 = 1.9

   LR(possible) = 240/444/300/556 = 0.54/0.54 = 1.0

   LR(unlikely) = 4/444/156/556 = 0.009/0.28 = 0.03.

2. The 2 × 2 table that corresponds to the Quick Test results according to the new "positive" and "negative" criteria is shown in Table 3.17.

   Sensitivity = a/(a + c) = 200/444 = 0.45 (45%)

   Specificity = d/(b + d) = 100/556 = 0.82 (82%)

   PPV = a/(a + b) = 200/300 = 0.67 (67%)

   NPV = d/(c + d) = 456/700 = 0.65 (65%).

TABLE 3.17   Quick Test Results and Disease Status

Quick Test	Disease Status +	Disease Status −	Total
+	200 (a)	100 (b)	300
−	244 (c)	456 (d)	700
Total	444	556	1000

3. The young woman's pretest probability of pneumonia is 75%. Her pretest odds are therefore $p/1 - p = 0.75/1 - 0.75 = 3/1$. Bayes theorem tells us that pretest odds $\times$ LR $=$ posttest odds. Since her chest X ray is normal, we use the negative LR of 0.6. The posttest odds are given by

$$3/1 \times 0.6 = 1.8.$$

We can convert these odds back to a probability:

Probability $=$ Odds in favor/Odds in favor $+$ Odds against $= 1.8/2.8$ $= 0.64 = 64\%$ (posttest probability).

An X ray was not warranted. The young woman's pretest probability is sufficiently high such that even a negative chest X ray result would not change management. In other words, with a 64% probability of pneumonia, the patient should be treated with antibiotics.

4. There are several major methodological problems with this study.

   i. The investigators studied "hospital employees" within a wide age range. These are not the type of people in which the diagnostic test would normally be employed.

   ii. The decision to obtain the confirmatory test was influenced by the new test's results. In other words, they should have obtained neurology consults on all patients, whether they tested positive on the oscillometer or not. After all, we do not know how many of those who tested negative have Parkinson disease!

   iii. The gold standard used was not appropriate. First it was not uniform, since four different neurologists were used. Second, these neurologists were already aware that the patients had tested positive on the oscillometer. This may have influenced their diagnosis. In general, clinical consultation is not a reliable enough gold standard for the diagnosis of disease, particularly when obtained from only one physician per patient.

5. This is an example of the *conjunction fallacy*. The patient certainly seems like someone likely to be having a heart attack (i.e., he is a prototypical heart attack patient). The probability of both not getting much exercise and having a heart attack, however, cannot be greater than the probability of either event alone. The correct answer, therefore is a.

6. We can begin by calculating sensitivity and specificity values for different cutoff points. For this purpose, 2 $\times$ 2 tables should be constructed (Tables 3.18–3.22).

TABLE 3.18   Cutoff of 10 or Greater

Lipase-beta Test Result	CF +	CF −
+	29	71
−	0	0
Total	29	71

Sensitivity $= 29/29 + 0 = 100\%$; specificity $= 0/71 + 0 = 0\%$.

TABLE 3.19   Cutoff of 20 or Greater

Lipase-beta Test Result	CF +	CF −
+	28	39
−	1	32
Total	29	71

Sensitivity $= 28/29 = 97\%$; specificity $= 32/71 = 45\%$.

TABLE 3.20   Cutoff of 30 or Greater

Lipase-beta Test Result	CF +	CF −
+	26	15
−	3	56
Total	29	71

Sensitivity $= 26/29 = 90\%$; specificity $= 79\%$.

TABLE 3.21   Cutoff of 40 or Greater

Lipase-beta Test Result	CF +	CF −
+	18	1
−	11	70
Total	29	71

Sensitivity $= 18/29 = 62\%$; specificity $= 70/71\% = 99\%$.

TABLE 3.22   Cutoff of 50 or Greater

Lipase-beta Test Result	CF +	CF −
+	10	1
−	19	70
Total	29	71

Sensitivity = 10/29 = 34%; specificity = 70/71% = 99%.

The best cutoff value is 30 μg/dL since it offers the best trade-off between sensitivity and specificity (i.e., both the sensitivity and specificity are reasonably high). A cutoff of 40 μg/dL also seems reasonable. We can also construct an ROC curve by plotting sensitivity against 1–specificity (Fig. 3.4).

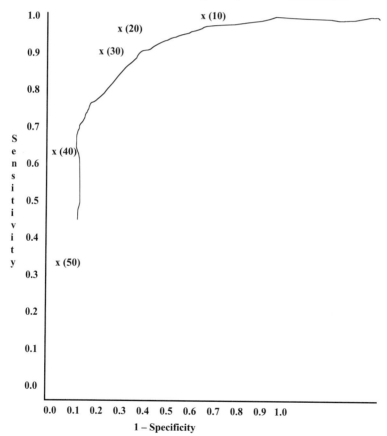

FIGURE 3.4 ROC Curve for Migraine Questionnaire Cutoffs

The cutoff of 30 μg/dL is closest to the top left corner of the graph. And therefore, according to the ROC curve, it is the best cutoff.

References

1. Pangaro L. A new vocabulary and other innovations for improving descriptive in-training evaluations. *Acad Med* 1999;74(11):1203–1207.
2. Elstein AS, Schwarz A. Clinical problem solving and diagnostic decision making: selective review of the cognitive literature. *Br Med J* 2002;324(7339): 729–732.
3. Price R. Essay towards solving a problem in the doctrine of chances. *Philos Trans R Soc Lond B Biol Sci* 1763; 53:370–418.
4. Economist.com. In praise of Bayes. URL: www.economist.com/displaystory. cfm?story_id=382968. Accessed May 30, 2005.
5. Kahneman's influence. URL: www.forensic-psych.com/artPrincetonWeekly 1.29.03.html. Accessed May 30, 2005.
6. Sackett DL, Haynes RB. The architecture of diagnostic research. *BMJ* 2002; 324(7336):539–541.

Design of Research to Evaluate Therapies

4

O B J E C T I V E S

1. List and describe five characteristics of a good clinical question.
2. Construct a precise clinical question that includes four essential elements.
3. Define the terms confounder, internal validity, and external validity.
4. Define the terms target population and accessible population.
5. Given a precise clinical question and a description of target and accessible populations, select inclusion and exclusion criteria for an appropriate study.
6. Distinguish between probability and nonprobability sampling.
7. Describe simple random sampling, stratified random sampling, cluster sampling, consecutive sampling, and convenience sampling.
8. Given a precise clinical question, define the null hypothesis and an alternate hypothesis for an appropriate study.
9. Define type 1 error and alpha, type 2 error and beta, and power.
10. Explain how the type 1 error rate, the magnitude of effect one is trying to detect in a study, and the sample size influence power.
11. Define noncentrality parameter.
12. In general terms, explain how the *critical value* can be used to derive a formula to estimate the sample size required for a study comparing two means of continuous data when the underlying populations are normally distributed.
13. Use a *rule of thumb* to estimate sample size for comparison of two means of continuous data when the underlying populations are normally distributed.
14. Define the term *bias*.
15. Define the term *randomization* and describe its purpose.
16. Define allocation and allocation concealment.
17. Describe simple randomization, block randomization, and stratified randomization.
18. Define the term *permutation*.
19. In the context of research to evaluate therapies, define the term *prognostic factor*.

101

4.1 Introduction

Physicians are more likely to encounter research about new therapies than any other kind in the medical literature. Research about new therapies certainly makes headlines both in the medical community and among the general public. New therapies are often thought of only as new medications. As discussed at the close of Chapter 10, a diagnostic test can be thought of as a new therapy when its impact upon specific outcomes is evaluated. Therapies can also take the form of counseling or advice, types of physical rehabilitation, surgeries or other invasive procedures, etc.

In general, the *randomized controlled trial* represents the best design for the evaluation of therapies. Different aspects of this design will be discussed in this chapter. The chapter takes the form of a story. The early history of the evaluation of therapies is followed by a scenario that forms the basis for a *step-wise* discussion of many important aspects of the design and evaluation of research about therapies. Some of these aspects are very complex. Only the bits most relevant to practicing physicians are discussed in depth.

4.2 Early History

Like the early history of diagnosis, for many centuries, the evaluation of therapies remained unscientific at best, and completely lacking at worst. The medieval practice of bloodletting by attaching leeches to the skin, for example, became a standard practice, not because it had been proven to work, but because it was consistent with spiritual beliefs about the causes of illness. Human history, however, does include some rare examples of efforts to make the evaluation of therapies rational and scientific. The Arab physician Avicenna (980–1037) laid down some simple rules for the evaluation of new drugs. He recommended, for example, that new drugs be studied in terms of their time of action and they should be studied more than once to find out if their effect is reproducible. Such forward thinking was scarce in much of the world for hundreds of years thereafter.

Scurvy, a disease caused by vitamin C deficiency, though uncommon today, was a common disease in the eighteenth century, especially among sailors. In 1747, a Scottish naval physician named James Lind decided to compare different treatments for scurvy. He took 12 sailors and divided them into 6 groups of 2. Each group of two received one of the following treatments: vinegar; seawater; elixir vitriol (diluted sulfuric acid); a mixture of garlic, mustard seeds, and Balsam of Peru; cider; or a combination of oranges and lemons. Lind carefully observed the sailors over a period of time and concluded that the oranges and lemons were best. Eventually, sailors brought along citrus fruit on long sea voyages to prevent scurvy. This is how English sailors became known as "limeys." Lind's work is more than an interesting story. He is often credited for having carried out the first *clinical trial*, an experimental approach comparing treatments among actual patients (as opposed to animals or lab specimens), which includes defined outcomes.

4.3 The Clinical Question

CASE 4.1

Atrial fibrillation is a relatively common disturbance of heart rhythm, which in addition to causing symptoms such as shortness of breath, is associated with an increased risk of stroke. To prevent stroke, patients with atrial fibrillation are usually given the blood thinner (anticoagulant) coumadin. Coumadin is effective in preventing stroke but is cumbersome to administer since it requires frequent monitoring of its effect. Your friend Jack has just invented a new drug he claims is more effective and safer than coumadin as an anticoagulant for the prevention of stroke among patients with atrial fibrillation. Furthermore, the new drug, Ceprotex, is easier to administer than coumadin. One regular dose given daily yields a more predictable "blood thinning" response. Patients can be safely given the medication without follow-up for several months. Your task is to determine the effectiveness of Ceprotex.

In the broadest sense, the purpose of research is to find answers to questions. Clinical research begins with development of one or more good clinical questions. You already likely have some idea of what constitutes a good clinical question. James Lind wanted to study different treatments for scurvy. This was important because scurvy was a serious disease at the time. It was a practical question to try to answer because different treatments were already being used, and a population at risk for scurvy (i.e., sailors) was readily available. The treatments Lind studied were relatively free of side effects. By contrast, consider an investigator who wishes to study the impact of zero gravity upon symptoms of migraine headache. This is not a rational question to answer for many reasons. It is, of course, impractical to place a significant number of migraine sufferers in a zero gravity environment.

Hulley and Cummings[1] have defined the characteristics of a good clinical question using the acronym FINER. A good clinical question should be *feasible*. Answering it should not require an impractically large number of subjects. The technical expertise to answer the question should be available. The research based on the question should not be too expensive, unmanageable, or time consuming. A good clinical question should be *interesting* to the investigator. Hulley and Cummings point out that researchers often have different motivations for pursuing clinical questions. Some, for example, are obliged to carry out research to support themselves financially. The best motivation for pursuing a clinical question is genuine curiosity about the answer. Good questions are also *novel*. This means they are designed to provide new, valuable information. Simply repeating a previous study using exactly same methods is often not worthwhile. Good questions are *ethical*. The research based on the question should not expose subjects to unacceptable risks and must always respect individual autonomy and privacy. Finally, and perhaps most importantly, clinical questions should be *relevant*. Consider again the question of migraine sufferers and zero gravity. Even if enough migraine sufferers could be placed in a zero gravity environment and the treatments were very effective, it is unlikely to be widely available to a large number of people. The impact of the study on the well-being of migraine sufferers, as a whole, therefore, would be minimal. In determining the relevance of a research question, list the possible outcomes of the research (e.g., treatment works; treatment does not work) and in each case ask yourself, "So what?" If you cannot come up with a good response, the question is probably irrelevant. Using the FINER criteria, let us return to the question of effectiveness of Ceprotex. Table 4.1 describes how such a question meets these general criteria.

TABLE 4.1   The Question of Effectiveness of Ceprotex

Feasible	Atrial fibrillation is common, and recruiting enough subjects should be easy. Technical expertise to carry out such research is widely available. Such research is expensive, but similar research has been done with other therapies. The resources, therefore, should be available.
Interesting	The question should be interesting to one or more investigators because atrial fibrillation is a serious problem for which the current treatment has drawbacks.
Novel	The question is novel since this therapy has not been previously evaluated.
Ethical	Such research can be carried out ethically, assuming that Ceprotex is as safe or safer than coumadin. The drug, therefore, would not expose patients to any greater risk than they would already experience using coumadin.
Relevant	The question is highly relevant since it would impact a large number of people and allow them to live a higher quality of life. The cumbersome monitoring that is necessary with coumadin would be avoided.

A good clinical question should certainly meet the FINER criteria, but what exactly is the question? Questions that are answerable are precise. Asking, "how effective is Ceprotex" is not precise enough. Sackett et al.[2] recommend a structured format for all clinical questions to make them as precise as possible. Four elements should be included. These include a specifically defined *patient* population or *problem*; an *intervention* (usually a treatment); a *comparison intervention* if necessary; and one or more precisely defined *outcomes*. These elements make up the acronym PICO.

Let us consider Ceprotex. In what types of patients and for what problems should it be studied? The drug is to be used to prevent stroke in patients with atrial fibrillation. Our patient population therefore consists only of patients with known atrial fibrillation. The intervention to be studied is Ceprotex. There are a couple of possible comparison interventions. We could compare Ceprotex to no specific drug treatment (e.g., compare Ceprotex to placebo). This would, however, be unethical. We know that coumadin prevents stroke. Not using any agent to prevent stroke in a group of patients exposes them to unreasonable risk. We should therefore compare Ceprotex to coumadin. The outcome we are interested in is stroke. Specifically, we wish to know if one drug prevents more strokes than the other. Stroke is an unfortunate medical event. The number of disease events occurring over a period of time is known as the incidence of disease. We say, for example, that "the 5-year incidence of myocardial infarction is 5%." This means 5% of patients will experience a myocardial infarction sometime within the 5 years. Five years is also a reasonable time frame for the incidence of stroke. Our outcome can be defined, therefore, as the *5-year incidence of stroke*.

We can now assemble our clinical question into the following form:

In patients with atrial fibrillation [P], is Ceprotex [I] or coumadin [C] associated with a lower 5-year incidence of stroke? [O]

The PICO format is widely used within the EBM paradigm and is a useful starting point in any clinical research.

4.4 Choosing Research Subjects

At first glance, the type of subjects that should be included in a study of Ceprotex seems fairly obvious: patients with atrial fibrillation. There are, however, a number of important additional considerations in recruiting people for the study. We wish to compare the effects of Ceprotex and coumadin on the incidence of stroke. Using an "idealistic" approach, we would like to recruit subjects that have atrial fibrillation and no other conditions, take no medications except for coumadin, are willing and able to participate in a study that will last 5 years, and have not had previous strokes (since people with previous strokes may be at especially high risk of future stroke). We would like to limit our recruitment to patients who meet these and similar criteria because we are only interested in the effect of the two medications on stroke, and wish to isolate this effect from other factors that may influence the incidence of stroke. For example, diabetes mellitus is a known risk factor for heart disease and stroke. Let us say we recruited patients with atrial fibrillation, without paying attention to which patients also had diabetes mellitus. Once the results of our study were obtained, it would be difficult to determine if any significant differences were due to the different medications, or if different rates and severities of diabetes in the treatment groups played a role. In this case, diabetes is a *confounder*—a factor that is associated with the variable or disease we are studying and also the outcome. In this case, many people with atrial fibrillation also have diabetes, and diabetes is associated with stroke. Diabetes among our study subjects makes it confusing to determine precisely the impact of the two medications upon stroke incidence. We can say that *diabetes* creates unwanted *noise* in our study that obscures the effect we are interested in. To minimize such noise, we try to limit our recruitment of subjects in such a way that the influence of confounders is minimized and so that any difference in stroke incidence can be attributable to the different medications. A study designed in a way that we can be sure that only the variables of interest influence the results is said to have *internal validity*.

Internal validity is important, but the preceding discussion hints at an important problem. Most patients with atrial fibrillation do not meet the ideal described previously. Most have some other condition, such as high blood pressure (a risk factor for stroke). Recruiting patients based on the ideal just discussed is therefore unrealistic. Furthermore, imagine that we did recruit patients who met the ideal and Ceprotex was found to be superior to coumadin. A physician reading the results might ask herself, "I do not have any patients like this in my practice. I wonder if Ceprotex would work as well among my patients with atrial fibrillation?" The drugs may behave in different ways among *typical* patients with atrial fibrillation. It is possible, for example, that the typical atrial fibrillation patient has so many other risk factors for stroke that any difference between Ceprotex and coumadin is relatively unimportant. The issue of whether or not the results of a study are applicable to different patients in other settings with the condition of interest is called the *generalizability* of the study. Generalizability is also referred to as *external validity*.

A good research study design delicately balances internal and external validity. By making recruitment too restrictive, external validity is jeopardized; by making recruitment too lax, internal validity is jeopardized. Keeping this principle in mind, the first step in deciding whom to study is to specify precisely the characteristics that study subjects must have. Patients with these characteristics are known as the *target population*. The target population must, of course, be selected on the basis of its ability to help answer the question of interest. There is no point, for example, in recruiting patients without atrial fibrillation into our study. Characteristics of our target population could include the following:

- Men and women aged 50 or older with diagnosed atrial fibrillation for at least 6 months. Age 50 or older is included to make the results more generalizable to the average patient with atrial fibrillation. "At least 6 months" is included because some patients have brief, transient episodes of atrial fibrillation and may be at lower risk of stroke than patients who have more chronic disease. This criterion was included to improve the internal validity of the study. Once the target population is defined, we can determine which of its members are *accessible* for study (accessible population). These include patients who live in a certain area or seek care in a particular institution or present with illness during a certain time. These characteristics of our patients address the practical or logistical aspects of recruitment. We could revise our study population to the following:
- Men and women aged 50 or older with diagnosed atrial fibrillation for at least 6 months who seek care at one or more of the University of Pittsburgh's teaching hospitals between January 1, 2007 and June 30, 2008. Using patients who seek care at teaching hospitals may be practical, since it is relatively easy to recruit subjects from and conduct research in such settings, but may threaten the generalizability of the results. Many patients with atrial fibrillation are cared for in community-based or primary care settings. It is known that patients in community settings differ from those who come to teaching hospitals in important ways. Depending upon the condition of interest, they are often less ill overall; in some cases, they are sicker. We could decide to recruit patients from community settings, but this may prove more time consuming and expensive.

The characteristics of the target and accessible populations are collectively known as the *inclusion criteria* for the study. *Exclusion criteria* describe patients who not only meet the inclusion criteria but also have conditions (i.e., confounders) that may influence the results by creating noise. These are specific conditions or characteristics patients should not have in order to participate in the study. Using too many exclusion criteria sacrifices the generalizability of the study. An appropriate list of exclusion criteria for our study could look like the following:

- no history of cancer of any kind
- no heart conditions other than atrial fibrillation
- must not be using drugs other than coumadin that are used to prevent stroke

Cancer may influence the risk of stroke, and perhaps more importantly, influences the chances that a patient will be able to participate in
a study that lasts for 5 years. Other heart conditions may influence the risk
of stroke. Simultaneously using other stroke preventive drugs obviously
makes it difficult to determine the effects of the drugs of interest. In most
studies, the list of inclusion and exclusion criteria is considerably longer
and more detailed. For the purpose of learning about research design, these
criteria are adequate.

4.5 Sampling

As discussed in Chapter 2, it is usually impractical to study all members of
a population. In Section 4.4, we discussed the possibility of using patients
with atrial fibrillation who are cared for in the teaching hospitals of one
city. All such patients constitute a population. There might be too many
patients to study. The process of selecting members of the accessible part
of the target population is known as *sampling*. There are two basic types of
sampling. *Probability sampling* uses techniques that ensure that each member of the population of interest has a known, specific chance of being selected for the study. In our case, for example, we could generate a list of
all patients with atrial fibrillation being cared for in teaching hospitals in
Pittsburgh. Let us say there are 1000 and each patient is assigned a number.
A computer could then be used to generate 100 random numbers between
1 and 1000. We could then use the random numbers to select the corresponding patients. This technique is known as *simple random sampling*.

Sometimes we are especially interested in the effect of a treatment upon
a specific group (e.g., women, African Americans, etc.). In such cases, we
can divide our population of interest into *strata* based upon such characteristics and then use simple random sampling within each stratum.
Let us say, for example, that we would like to recruit equal numbers of
European and African Americans into our Ceprotex study but there are far
fewer African Americans among atrial fibrillation patients in Pittsburgh's
teaching hospitals. If we used simple random sampling, there would be
few African Americans enrolled in the study. We can get around this problem by dividing the population of interest by race and then using simple random sampling in each population until we have recruited roughly
equal numbers of each group. This technique is known as *stratified random
sampling*.

Cluster sampling takes advantage of natural groupings of patients and is
useful when the population of interest is spread out geographically. Let us
say, for example, that our population of interest was not limited to teaching hospitals in Pittsburgh but to all teaching hospitals in the United States.
To list all atrial fibrillation patients in all teaching hospitals in the United
States and then select a number of patients at random would be difficult.

Alternatively, we could list all the teaching hospitals in the United States and then select a certain number of *these* at random. We could then randomly select patients from within these randomly selected hospitals. There are, therefore, two levels of random selection.

Nonprobability sampling does not use such methods to randomly select study subjects and is often easier and less expensive than probability sampling. Two popular methods include *consecutive* and *convenience sampling*. Consecutive sampling involves simply trying to recruit every patient who meets the inclusion and exclusion criteria over a certain period of time. In our case, we could simply ask every patient with atrial fibrillation who comes to one of the teaching hospitals during the study period to participate until we had recruited an adequate number. Convenience sampling is the method of taking patients who are most readily available. In our case, for example, suppose 100 patients with atrial fibrillation just happen to be attending a conference about good nutrition. Recruiting this sample of patients would clearly be very convenient! A more realistic convenience sample would be all patients in one teaching hospital *currently* on a list of atrial fibrillation patients.

What type of sampling should we use? A consecutive sample is appropriate unless it is too large. In other words, it is appropriate unless too many atrial fibrillation patients are seen in teaching hospitals during the study period. In such cases, we could use a simple random sample of all such patients. Let us assume for this case that we are not especially interested in any specific stratum of the population of interest. Cluster sampling is unnecessary in our case since the number of teaching hospitals and the total number of patients is probably not too large. Let us assume that a truly *convenient* sample is unavailable.

4.6 Defining Outcomes

We have defined the type (though not the number) of patients we wish to study. What precisely do we wish to measure? In our case, the major outcome has already been defined: 5-year incidence of stroke. We will follow patients enrolled in the study over the course of 5 years and determine if they have a stroke at any point in the 5-year period. The outcome, therefore, could take a simple "yes" (i.e., did have a stroke) or "no" *categorical* form. It is possible that some patients may experience more than one stroke over the 5-year period. We could record each stroke as a "yes" and then compare the number of strokes among patients on each drug. In this case, our outcome is therefore the total number of strokes in each treatment group, rather than the total number of patients experiencing one or more strokes. Let us use this outcome for our study. Since it is the main outcome we are interested in, it is known as our *principal outcome*.

In addition to our principal outcome, we may be interested in other outcomes. For example, we may be interested in the number of heart attacks that occur with each drug. If Ceprotex reduces the incidence of stroke but also substantially increases the incidence of heart attack, it may not be a very useful new drug. It is possible, for whatever reason, that despite a reduction in the incidence of stroke, Ceprotex is associated with more deaths. A common side effect of medications designed to protect against stroke is gastrointestinal (GI) bleeding. We may wish to measure the 5-year incidence of GI bleeding in patients on Ceprotex and coumadin. Outcomes other than the principal outcome under study, such as the incidence of GI bleeding, are known as *secondary outcomes.*

4.7 Formulating Hypotheses

Hypotheses are necessary in any study in which tests of statistical significance such as those discussed in Chapter 2 are used. A hypothesis is a theory about what might be found in a study. For Case 4.1, for example, one hypothesis might be that Ceprotex is superior to coumadin in preventing stroke. Another might be that Ceprotex is worse than coumadin in preventing stroke. Still another possible hypothesis is that Ceprotex is neither worse nor any better than coumadin in preventing stroke (i.e., the two therapies are equivalent). This last hypothesis is especially important in the evaluation of therapies. Recall that the statistical tests we discussed in Chapter 2 yielded significant values if two or more sets of data differed by a degree that was unlikely to occur by chance. The tests of significance use the assumption that two or more sets of data are equivalent. The actual values of the test are compared to values that would have occurred had the sets of data actually been equivalent. For the Wilcoxan rank sum test, for example, we compare the value of W to all possible values of rank sums that could occur assuming that the treatments being compared are equivalent. This assumption is rejected if the value of the test falls outside a prespecified level of significance (usually 0.05).

The assumption of equivalence is known as the *null hypothesis* (H_o). In designing a study to evaluate two therapies, we begin with the null hypothesis and then specify the conditions under which we will either reject it (i.e., find that the therapies are not equivalent) or accept it (find that the therapies are equivalent). For Case 4.1, the null hypothesis can be stated as the following:

H_o = Among patients with atrial fibrillation, there is *no* difference between the effects of Ceprotex and coumadin upon the 5-year incidence of stroke.

Notice that the null hypothesis includes the four elements of our clinical question. Hypotheses other than the null hypothesis are known as *alternate hypotheses*. A simple alternate hypothesis includes the following:

H_1 = Among patients with atrial fibrillation, there *is* a difference between the effects of Ceprotex and coumadin upon the 5-year incidence of stroke.

There are actually an infinite number of alternate hypotheses, e.g., "Ceprotex is twice as effective as coumadin in preventing stroke," "Ceprotex is 5% less effective that coumadin in preventing stroke," etc. The conventional design of a clinical trial only allows us to collect enough evidence to accept or reject the null hypothesis with a reasonable degree of certainty. If we do reject the null hypothesis, we can conclude that the two therapies are not equivalent (i.e., consistent with the general alternate hypothesis of nonequivalence) but we will not know how likely each of the infinite number of alternate hypotheses is.

To evaluate the effectiveness of Ceprotex, we will recruit a sample of patients and based on our results, draw conclusions about the effectiveness of this new drug among the entire population of patients with atrial fibrillation (i.e., statistical inference). Our conclusion based on a test of significance may be wrong. Recall that with statistical tests, we accept a value as statistically significant if the chances of getting that value or a more extreme value is less than a prespecified level, usually 5% or less, under the assumption that two sets of data are equivalent. Therefore, there is still the possibility that our conclusion based on a test of significance, although unlikely, is wrong. Let us say we obtain a value for a t test, for example, and a value as extreme as or more extreme than this value has a 4% chance of occurring when two groups being compared are equivalent. If we conclude that the two groups are not equivalent based on such a t test result, we would still be wrong 4% of the time. We can never be 100% correct and must specify the level of significance we are willing to accept before concluding that the two groups being compared are different. Similarly, in studies of therapy, there is the possibility of rejecting the null hypothesis (i.e., finding that two treatments are not equivalent) even though two treatments are equivalent. There is also the possibility of accepting the null hypothesis (i.e., finding that two treatments are equivalent) even though the two treatments are not equivalent. In both cases we will have committed an error.

Rejecting the null hypothesis when two treatments are actually equivalent (i.e., the null hypothesis is true) is known as a *type 1 error*. Accepting the null hypothesis when two treatments are not equivalent (i.e., the null hypothesis is false) is known as a *type 2 error*. When we performed tests of significance in Chapter 2, we always specified a level of significance at which we would reject the assumption that two sets of data are equivalent. Similarly, in the design of a study of two therapies, we need to specify the rates of type 1 and type 2 error we are willing to accept when we make

TABLE 4.2   Conclusions About Null Hypothesis and Possible Errors

Our action based on the results of our study	Truth in the Population	
	Two treatments are not equivalent	Two treatments are equivalent
Reject null hypothesis	Correct Decision	Type 1 Error
Accept null hypothesis	Type 2 Error	Correct Decision

conclusions about the null hypothesis. The maximum type 1 error rate we are willing to accept is known as alpha (α). The maximum type 2 error rate we are willing to accept is known as beta (β). The 2 × 2 table (Table 4.2) summarizes our possible conclusions about the null hypothesis based on the results from our *sample* and the possible errors that could result when what is actually true in the *population* differs from our conclusions.

Researchers specify α and β in the design phase of the study and use these values when they analyze data at the end of a study. For example, upon completion of a study, the difference between two treatments could be analyzed using a statistical test of significance. If it was found that the value of the test of significance or a value more extreme would occur only 3% of the time, assuming that the two treatments are equivalent and the prespecified α was 0.05, one would reject the null hypothesis.

This α and β can be described in words that make them easier to conceptualize. α is:

the chance we are willing to accept of being wrong by finding a difference between two treatments when none really exists.

β is:

the chance we are willing to accept of being wrong by not finding a difference between two treatments when there really is a difference.

If there really is a difference between two treatments, our study can be designed to either find it or not find it. If β is the chance of not finding it, it makes sense that $1 - \beta$ is the chance of finding it. This $1 - \beta$ is an important quantity known as the *power* of a study. Power is defined as the chance of finding a difference between treatments based on the sample studied when one really does exist in the population. Power is especially important when interpreting the results of a study that concludes that there is no difference between treatments. If the study was designed with a low power, an important difference between treatments may have been missed.

Usually α is set at 0.05 and β at 0.20. The levels, however, should be set according to the question addressed by the study and the study's priorities. Consider the case of a new therapy that has just come out on the market for relief of fever. It is compared to an existing therapy for fever that has been around for many years which, overall, is both effective and safe. In such cases, we would want to be especially careful to avoid finding a difference between the treatments when one does not exist (type 1 error). This is because if we made a type 2 error, the only consequence would be that people would continue to use the older, effective treatment for fever. On the other hand, if we made a type 1 error, people would likely switch to the new therapy unnecessarily. We would like to keep α low in this case. By contrast, consider the case of a new therapy for a terminal illness. An existing treatment is of little or no benefit to patients. In such a case, we would be less concerned with the type 1 error rate and more concerned with minimizing the type 2 error rate. We *want* to find any possible difference between the new and old therapies if one exists. The only consequence of making a type 1 error in this situation is that people would switch to the new therapy from an old therapy that was ineffective. The consequence of a type 2 error, by contrast, is that people would not benefit from a potentially life-saving therapy.

4.8 Determinants of Power

In the design phase of a study, α and power are two important values that are usually set . There are several important factors that determine the power of a study (Table 4.3). It is possible to adjust or fix these factors at prespecified values and then determine the power that would result. Alternatively, we could determine the power we would like to achieve and then adjust the other factors accordingly. In either case, understanding the determinants of power is crucial. The power of a study depends upon three interdependent factors:

TABLE 4.3   Factors Influencing the Power of a Study

Type 1 Error Rate (α)	The smaller the desired α in the design of a study, the lower is the power of the study.
Noncentrality parameter	The larger the ratio of the magnitude of the effect one is trying to detect to the standard deviation of the outcome variable in the population, the higher is the power of the study.
Sample size	The larger the sample size of a study, the higher is its power.

- The type 1 error rate (α),
- The size of the difference you wish to detect between treatments relative to the amount of variability in the outcome variable in the population,
- The number of subjects in each group being compared (known as the *sample size*).

Rather than providing mathematical proofs for why these factors determine power, let us follow an intuitive approach. First, the type 1 error rate is the risk that we will reject the null hypothesis incorrectly and conclude that there is a difference between the groups being compared. Therefore, α is the risk of finding a difference when there is not one. If we set α to a very small value, we would be very sure of not making the mistake of finding a difference when one does not exist. There is a price to pay for being so certain of not making this mistake. By making sure we do not mistakenly find a difference when one does not exist, it makes sense that we are sacrificing our ability to find a difference when one does exist.

Consider this analogy: The victim of a robbery provides the police with a very detailed description through memory of a perpetrator, including hair color, eyes, height, build, etc. In seeking suspects for the case, if the police rounded up only men who *exactly* fit the description, they would be sure not to make the mistake of catching someone who is innocent (equivalent to avoiding a type 1 error). On the other hand, it becomes more likely that they would miss the perpetrator entirely, since he may be someone who does not entirely fit the description (equivalent to committing a type 2 error). Similarly, by keeping α low, we sacrifice the power to find a difference. The lower is the level of α, therefore, the higher is the level of β, and the lower is the power since power $= 1 - \beta$.

It is easier to detect big differences between groups being compared than small differences. This should be intuitively obvious. Imagine a group of 10 men, all of whom are between 6′ and 6′3″ tall. Imagine another group of 10 men, all of whom are between 5′4″ and 5′7″ tall. If these two groups stood next to each other, it would be very easy to tell which group was taller. Alternatively, imagine a group of 10 men between 5′10″ and 6′ tall and another between 5′9″ and 5′11″ tall. Detecting this smaller difference between the two groups is much harder. You, therefore, would have *less power* to detect a smaller difference. When we design a study, we decide upon the *magnitude of effect* that we wish to detect. This is usually the smallest magnitude of effect we consider to be clinically important. Imagine in Case 4.1, for example, that it turns out that Ceprotex is associated with 15 fewer strokes per 1000 people than coumadin over a 5-year period. This is a significant difference between the two treatments. Such a difference would likely persuade many physicians to prescribe Ceprotex instead of coumadin. Alternatively, imagine that the difference turns out to be much smaller, such as 4 per 1000. This difference may be clinically unimportant. We may decide in the design phase of the study that a difference smaller than 10 (per 1000) is not worth detecting, since it would not change how patients are managed. Therefore, there would be no point, under those circumstances, to design a study with the power to detect differences smaller than 10. The magnitude of effect we wish to detect is usually designated by the Greek symbol for delta (δ).

The power to detect differences between groups is influenced not only by the absolute magnitude of effect we wish to detect, but also the ratio of this magnitude to the amount of variability of the outcome variable in the population we are studying. Imagine that we are studying the impact of two drugs upon the blood sugar of patients in two different populations of diabetics. In the first population being studied, let us say blood sugar values all cluster tightly in a range of 115–125 mg/dL. In the second population, let us say blood sugar values are more variable, with a range of 90–200 mg/dL. Now let us say that the difference in the two treatments we wish to detect is 50 mg/dL. In which of the two populations would a difference of this magnitude be easier to detect? In the second population, such a difference could easily get *lost* because blood sugar is so variable. The difference would be easier to detect in the first population. The power of a study, therefore, depends upon the ratio of the magnitude of effect to the variability of the outcome variable in the population as represented by its standard deviation (σ). This ratio is known as a *noncentrality parameter* and represented by the Greek symbol for phi (Φ).

$$\Phi = \delta/\sigma.$$

Larger values of phi are easier to detect and associated with higher power.

The larger the sample size of a study, the higher is the study's power. This makes intuitive sense. The larger a sample is, the more it resembles the population from which it was drawn and the less likely we are to make errors in statistical inference (i.e., lower α and lower β). The relationship of power to sample size is an important one. In the design phase of a study, instead of setting a specific sample size and calculating the resulting power, researchers usually start with a prespecified value of power and then determine the sample size needed to achieve it. Estimating sample size is discussed in the next section.

4.9 Determining Sample Size

To physicians, one of the most mysterious aspects of the design of studies of therapy is determining sample size. Power, the type 1 error rate, the relative magnitude of effect one wishes to detect, and sample size are all intrinsically linked. As a general principle, the surer one wants to be that the conclusions of a clinical study represent the truth in the population, the more study subjects (i.e., larger sample size) that are needed. This means that both higher power and lower α require larger sample sizes. The smaller the magnitude of effect one wants to detect in relation to the standard deviation of the outcome variable, the larger the sample size required. While these general relationships are intuitively obvious, calculating precise numbers of subjects required for a study can get complicated. The approach differs according to what type of outcome is being measured (e.g., continuous, dichotomous).

Let us consider one common situation, the sample size required for the comparison of two means when the outcome is measured on a continuous scale and is normally distributed. Let us say we wish to compare the effect of two different blood pressure lowering medications, A and B. Let us assume that the absolute magnitude of effect upon systolic blood pressure that we feel is worth detecting is 10 mmHg (δ). There are three additional values that we need to specify in order to calculate sample size: α, β, and the standard deviation of the outcome variable in the population. Notice that we have split the noncentrality parameter into its two constituents (δ and σ). This split will be temporary. Let us say we wish α to be 0.05 and β to be 0.20 (i.e., power of 80%). Let us also say that we know from previous studies that σ of systolic blood pressure in the general population is 20 mmgHg. To begin to understand how sample size is calculated, take a look at Fig. 4.1.

The figure looks intimidating, but will become clear as we dissect it. This requires a bit of math and logic. Working through it, however, will take some of the mystery out of estimating sample size. First, we said that we are designing a study to compare two means of a continuous outcome that is normally distributed. There are two possible conclusions from our study: The null hypothesis (H_o) is true (i.e., treatments are equivalent) or the null hypothesis is false (i.e., the treatments are different). The curves in Fig. 4.1 represent plots of the possible *differences* between the mean blood pressure with drug A and B, under these two different circumstances. The curve on the left is drawn assuming the null hypothesis is true, that is, there is no significant difference in systolic blood pressure between drugs A and B. Notice that this curve centers around a difference of zero. This makes sense. If we assume the null hypothesis is true, the most frequent difference to occur under that assumption should be no difference.

The curve on the right represents the differences between the mean blood pressure with drug A and drug B assuming that there is a difference in means equivalent to the magnitude of effect we specified (δ). We decided

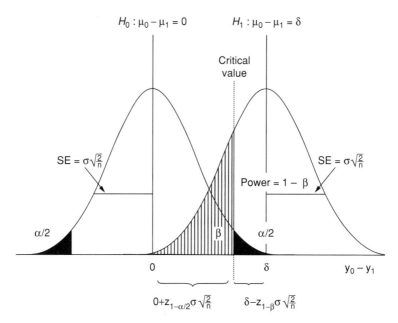

FIGURE 4.1 Graphical Model for Illustrating Sample Size Calculations

Reproduced with permission from van Belle G. Statistical Rules of Thumb. Hoboken, NJ, Wiley-Interscience; 2002, p. 30.)

this was 10 mmHg. The curve is shifted rightward and centers around the difference of δ. Once again, this makes sense. If we assume that the difference in mean blood pressure between drugs A and B is 10 mmHg, this is the most frequent difference we would find under that assumption.

Notice that the two curves overlap to some extent. It is in this overlap that we could make type 1 or type 2 errors. The critical value is the value at which we either reject or accept the null hypothesis. If we find a mean difference that falls to the left of the critical value, we would accept the null hypothesis. Clearly there is a risk of being wrong, represented by the shaded area β. On the other hand, if we find a mean difference to the right of the critical value, we would reject the null hypothesis. The risk of being wrong is represented by the shaded area $\alpha/2$. We use $\alpha/2$ rather than α because it is the $\alpha/2$ portion of the left curve that is to the right of the critical value.

Suppose we wish to detect a larger magnitude of effect. In your mind, you can imagine that the right hand curve would move rightward. Under those circumstances, the area shaded for β would decrease in size (i.e., power increases). Similarly, if we wish to detect a smaller magnitude of effect, the right hand curve would move to the left and there would be more overlap between the two curves. The area shaded for β would increase in size (i.e., power decreases). This is a graphical explanation for how power is influenced by magnitude of effect.

We have two plots of differences of sample means. In Chapter 2, we learned that the standard error of the difference of two means is given by

$$(SEM)^2_{\overline{O}-\overline{U}} = (SEM)^2_{\overline{O}} + (SEM)^2_{\overline{U}},$$

where $\overline{O}$ and $\overline{U}$ are variables representing the means of two different samples.

Recall that SEM^2 can also be represented by

$$(SEM)^2 = s^2_{\overline{O}}/n_{\overline{O}} + s^2_{\overline{U}}/n_{\overline{U}},$$

where $s^2_{\overline{O}}$ and $s^2_{\overline{U}}$ are the variances of the two samples, and $n_{\overline{O}}$ and $n_{\overline{U}}$ are the sizes of the two samples. For the purpose of calculating sample size, we can assume that the sample will be the same size whether or not the null hypothesis is true. We can also use our estimate of the population variance in place of variances of different samples, whether or not the null hypothesis is true. In our case,

$$SEM^2 \text{ (differences in blood pressure)} = \sigma^2/n + \sigma^2/n = 2 \times (\sigma^2/n).$$

Therefore,

$$SEM \text{ (differences in blood pressure)} = \sigma \times \sqrt{2/n}.$$

Now, let us express the critical value in Fig. 4.1 in two different ways. In the left hand curve, the critical value occurs at $\alpha/2$. This point can be expressed as the mean of the curve plus the number of standard errors above the mean that corresponds to $\alpha/2$. The number of standard errors above the mean can be expressed using z scores. Specifically, we need the z score that corresponds to $1 - \alpha/2$, i.e., $z_{(1-\alpha/2)}$ is the number of standard errors above the mean for the location of the critical value in the left hand curve. To find the actual value that corresponds to this z score, we need to multiply it by the SEM (differences in blood pressure).

Our critical value can therefore be expressed as

$$0 + z_{1-\alpha/2} \times \sigma \times \sqrt{2/n}.$$

Now, let us express the critical value using the curve on the right. Here the critical value is to the left of δ. Specifically, it is $(1 - \beta)z$ scores to the left of δ. We can now express the critical value as

$$\delta - z_{1-\beta} \times \sigma\sqrt{2/n}.$$

These two expressions must be equal.

$$0 + z_{1-\alpha/2} \times [\sigma\sqrt{2/n}] = \delta - z_{1-\beta} \times [\sigma\sqrt{2/n}].$$

Solving for n, we find

$$n = \frac{2(z_{1-\alpha/2} + z_{1-\beta})^2}{(\delta/\sigma)^2}.$$

Notice that the denominator is the square of the noncentrality parameter. Let us return to our blood pressure example. For $\alpha = 0.05$ and $\beta = 0.20$, $z_{1-\alpha/2}$ and $z_{1-\beta}$ are 1.96 and 0.84, respectively.

$$2(z_{1-\alpha/2} + z_{1-\beta})^2 = 15.68 \text{ (or roughly 16)}.$$

Our δ is 10 and σ is 20. The denominator is therefore 0.25. Therefore, n is roughly 64 subjects per group.

Let us return to the example of Case 4.1. Let us once again use α of 0.05 and β of 0.2. The numerator in our equation to estimate sample size, therefore, remains 16. Let us say the magnitude of effect we wish to detect is still a difference of 10 in 5-year incidence/1000. Let us assume that the standard deviation of the incidence of strokes in the population corresponds to roughly 14. Our estimate of sample size is therefore,

$$n = 16/(10/14)^2 = 31 \text{ (approximately)}.$$

Roughly 31 subjects per each of the two groups are required for Jack's study. This is the number that is required at the end of the study for analysis. This does not take into consideration *drop outs*, those who choose to discontinue a study prior to completion for whatever reason. Subjects may also die unexpectedly, move away, etc. According to our sample size calculation, we would only need to recruit a total of 62 subjects (31 × 2 groups) for the study. Because of the phenomenon of drop outs and other reasons for loss of study subjects prior to completion, it would be wise to recruit significantly more than this number. Clinical trials often recruit 20% more subjects or greater to compensate for subjects lost during the course of the study. For Jack's study, recruiting a total of 100 subjects is reasonable.

Since α of 0.05 and β of 0.20 are very commonly used in the design of studies of therapies, the numerator in our two sample size calculations thus far provides a useful rule of thumb for determining the sample size required for the comparison of two means of continuous data when underlying population is assumed to be normally distributed.

Rule of thumb: $n = 16/(\phi)^2$.

4.10 Allocation

Allocation is the process by which a patient receives one treatment or another in a clinical trial. The way treatments are allocated is extremely important. Imagine that for Jack's study, the healthiest 50% of the subjects we recruited receive Ceprotex, and the remainder receive coumadin. Clearly, this is an unfair comparison. If we found at the end of the trial that Ceprotex prevented more strokes than coumadin we would be left wondering whether the results were due to Ceprotex or the comparatively good health of the study subjects who received it. As noted, the *randomized controlled trial* is usually the best way to study new therapies. This design has some extremely important features. Designing a good study of therapies requires not only careful planning in recruitment, determining sample size, etc., but also making sure that the study is not prone to a phenomenon called *bias*.

Bias is a systematic error in the way a study is carried out that can lead to false conclusions. If we did assign the healthiest 50% of patients to Ceprotex and found that Ceprotex was more effective in reducing the incidence of stroke, this would not be a correct conclusion, since the way subjects were allocated to treatment was *biased*. The emergence of a *confounding variable* or *confounder* is one mechanism through which bias influences the result of a study. Let us say that we decide to recruit patients for our Ceprotex study from two different nursing homes. One is a private nursing facility; the other, a government run facility. Let us say we decide to give Ceprotex to all the recruits from the private facility and coumadin to the others. Let us also say that it turns out that the patients in the private facility take a higher average number of medications than the patients in the government facility. Many medications can interfere with both Ceprotex and coumadin. In this case, the bias is allocating treatment based on nursing home facility. The resulting confounder is the number of medications each patient takes, which differs significantly between nursing homes.

Randomization is a method based on chance that is the preferred way to allocate treatments. In a randomized trial, each patient has an equal chance of receiving either of the treatments being compared. The purpose of randomization is to minimize bias and make sure that the two groups being compared are as similar as possible. Randomization is useful in creating two groups that are similar with respect to common factors like age, sex, and race. It is not usually possible in advance to identify all possible confounders—the underlying variables that might influence the outcome. Randomization, however, can be used to distribute confounders equally between the groups being compared. Take our aforementioned example of patients from the two different nursing homes. Even if we did not know that the number of previous medications being taken could influence the outcome, through randomization, every patient, regardless of which nursing home he lived in, would have an equal chance of receiving either Ceprotex or coumadin. Under such a scheme, each of the two treatment groups is likely to have a roughly equal number of subjects taking lots of medications and few medications.

Blinding is a deliberate process whereby study subjects and/or investigators are kept ignorant of the treatment allocation of each patient. Like randomization, its purpose is to reduce bias. In a single-blind study, patients are unaware of which treatment they are receiving. In Jack's study, for example, this would involve making sure that patients could not tell whether they were taking coumadin or Ceprotex. Blinding subjects to treatment in this fashion can be complicated and involves, for example, making sure that the two pills look alike. It is not difficult to imagine how bias could result if patients knew which pill they were taking. The patients taking the new pill may be less likely to report symptoms of very minor strokes, for example, because they may be confident that the new treatment is superior. In a double-blind study, both the patients and the investigators carrying out the study are blinded to treatment allocation. An investigator keen to prove the superiority of Ceprotex may treat patients assigned to the Ceprotex group differently from patients assigned to the coumadin group. This could bias the results of the study. In a triple-blind study, the patients, investigators, and those who measure the outcome of the study are unaware of the treatment assignment. Let us say, for example, that patients and investigators are unaware of which patients received Ceprotex but the neurologist who determines whether a patient had a stroke is aware of the treatment allocation. He may have some conscious or subconscious bias against either Ceprotex or coumadin that could influence his diagnosis.

Allocation concealment refers to keeping those responsible for recruiting patients unaware of the randomization scheme by which patients are assigned to one treatment or another. This prevents recruiters from selecting patients for study, whom they feel should be in one group or another. Let us say that our study uses a very simplistic randomization scheme: The first patient recruited is assigned to Ceprotex, the next to coumadin, the third to Ceprotex, the fourth to coumadin, and so on. If recruiters are aware of this scheme, they would easily be able to figure out to which treatment the next patient will be assigned. They may try to recruit patients with particular characteristics to one group or the other.

There are several ways to randomize participants to one treatment or another. *Simple randomization* is like flipping a coin. For example, if the coin comes up heads, the patient receives Ceprotex; if it comes up tails, the patient receives coumadin. In reality, researchers use tables of random numbers or random number generators rather than coins for simple randomization. Imagine that we successfully recruit 100 patients into our Ceprotex trial and assign each a unique number from 1 to 100. Now, let us say we have a computer program that generates random numbers between 1 and

100 and the program does not provide the same number twice. Let us say the program is run once and spits out the number 8. The patient assigned to the number 8 could receive Ceprotex. If on the next run, the program spits out 43, the patient assigned to number 43 could receive coumadin. We could alternate treatment assignment in this fashion until all the numbers are exhausted.

In very large studies, through simple randomization, the number of patients assigned to each of the two treatments should be very close to equal. In smaller studies, however, it is possible through simple randomization for significantly more patients to be assigned to one treatment than another. This has negative consequences. The more unequal the number of patients assigned to each treatment group, the lower is the power of the study. To make sure that the two groups are balanced in terms of size, *block randomization* is used. In this method, *blocks* of patients are randomized according to a balanced sequence whose order changes in each block. Let us say that we wish to randomize blocks of four patients to one of two treatments, A or B. Our block sequence could be

ABBA.

Notice that the number of patients assigned to each treatment (A or B) is balanced at two each. For another block, the sequence could be

BBAA.

Once again, the block of four patients is balanced. It is the sequence of treatment assignment that varies from block to block. How are these block sequences selected? Each sequence is known as a *permutation*—simply one possible way the same set of numbers can be ordered. With a block size of four, and two possible treatments, there are a total of six possible permutations:

AABB

ABAB

ABBA

BBAA

BABA

BAAB

One possible way to select a sequence for each block is to assign a number (1–6) to each permutation and then use a program that generates random numbers between 1 and 6 to select the sequence for each block of four new patients who are recruited.

As discussed, a confounder is a variable other than the variable under study that influences the outcome. It is usually unknown to us at the outset of a study. When we suspect that a variable does influence the outcome of a study, it is important to measure subjects with respect to this variable before applying the interventions. In our Ceprotex study, for example, we may suspect that sex, age, systolic blood pressure, or other factors could influence the incidence of stroke. Such variables are known as *prognostic factors*. Recall that one of the purposes of randomization is to create groups that are as equal as possible. If we are concerned that through simple randomization, groups might be imbalanced with respect to one or more prognostic factors, we can use a procedure known as *stratified randomization*. Let us say that we believe that age and sex influence the incidence of stroke. Specifically, we would like to divide the participants by age into two categories: age 60 and over, and age less than 60. Combining sex and these age categories, we have four strata:

Male, age < 60

Male, age ≥ 60

Female, age < 60

Female, age ≥ 60

We now randomize patients within each stratum, using block randomization as discussed before or some other method:

Male, age < 60 AABB, ABAB, etc.

Male, age ≥ 60 ABBA, BAAB, etc.

Female, age < 60 BABA, AABB, etc.

Female, age ≥ 60 BBAA, ABAB, etc.

We now have the essential tools to design a study to evaluate Ceprotex. We have defined a precise question, developed hypotheses, and determined the conditions under which we will accept or reject the null hypothesis. We have estimated the number of subjects we will need (roughly 31 for each group, though 50 per group would be a safer number given possible drop outs). We can use simple randomization to allocate patients to each group, but to keep the groups balanced, it would be wiser to use block randomization. If we are concerned about the influence of certain prognostic factors, we can randomize patients by strata such as age, sex, and presence of other conditions. Patients in each stratum can be assigned to a treatment using block randomization.

PROBLEMS

1. Diabetes is treated with insulin. Oralin is a new form of insulin that can be taken "orally" without being broken down in the digestive tract, and therefore avoiding the cumbersome injections needed with conventional insulin. Its manufacturer claims that use of Oralin twice daily can achieve glucose control as good if not better than conventional insulin, as measured by lower mean fasting glucose levels in patients with type I diabetes. Using this information, construct a sound "answerable" clinical question that can form the basis of a study of Oralin.

2. Construct a null and general alternative hypothesis based on the study for which you constructed a sound clinical question in Problem 1.

3. Two different behavioral therapies for smoking cessation are being compared in a clinical trial. Participants receiving therapy A were all male subjects from a veterans' hospital outpatient clinic. Participants receiving therapy B were all male subjects recruited by placing an ad in a newspaper. In what way(s) could the results of this study be biased based upon this recruitment strategy?

4. You are interested in designing a trial comparing two treatments for antibiotic treatments (A and B) for community-acquired pneumonia. The principal outcome is "number of days until complete relief of symptoms," and is normally distributed. The standard deviation of the number of days until complete relief among patients with community-acquired pneumonia is 2 days. Approximately how many patients would you like to enroll in the study, assuming that the smallest difference in mean magnitude of effect worth detecting is 1 day and assuming you want 80% power and a maximum type 1 error rate of 5%? How does the number of enrollees change assuming you want 90% power with the same type 1 error rate and magnitude of effect?

5. A clinical trial has been designed to measure the impact of a new drug for HIV designed to boost CD4 cell counts. CD4 cell counts are a measure of the degree of imune system impairment. CD4 counts are measured on a continuous scale and are normally distributed in the population of HIV patients. The new drug is being compared to a placebo drug. The trial has been designed to detect a difference in mean CD4 counts between the new drug and placebo groups of 20. The standard deviation of CD4 count in the HIV population is 25. The acceptable

type 1 error rate has been set at 0.05. It has been a struggle to recruit patients to the study. So far, a total of 80 patients have been recruited. What is the maximum power of the study if it was to begin today and all 80 recruits participated?

6. A trial is being designed to compare two different treatments for influenza. It is extremely important to have equal number of subjects in each of the two treatment groups. Recruitment for the study is difficult and unpredictable. At a certain point, the flu season ends and it will not be possible to recruit any more subjects. Block randomization is being used with block size of six patients. What is the maximum possible difference in the size of the two groups at the end of recruitment under such a randomization scheme and why?

SOLUTIONS TO PROBLEMS

1. A good clinical question includes four elements: (1) patient or problem; (2) intervention; (3) a comparison intervention if applicable; and (4) an outcome. An appropriate clinical question would be the following:

   In patients with type 1 diabetes, can Oralin therapy, as opposed to conventional insulin, achieve glucose control that is as good or better as measured by mean fasting glucose.

2. The null hypothesis based upon the clinical question in Problem 1 would be the following:

   H_o = *There is no statistically significant difference in the effects of Oralin and conventional insulin upon mean fasting glucose.*

   H_1 = *There is a statistically significant difference in the effects of Oralin and conventional insulin upon mean fasting glucose.*

3. Male patients from a veterans' hospital are likely to be older than those recruited through an ad placed in a newspaper. Such older patients may be smokers for much longer than other patients. It may be harder for patients with a longer smoking history to quit smoking. The results of the study may reveal, therefore, that therapy A is less effective than therapy B. It would be hard to determine if such a difference is due to the therapy or the difference in the two groups being compared. Duration of smoking and age might *confound* the results.

4. We can use our rule of thumb to answer the first question about sample size, whereby $n = 16/\phi^2$. With 80% power, $\alpha = 0.05$, a magnitude of effect of 1 day, and a standard deviation of 2 days,

$$n = 16/(1/2)^2 = 64.$$

Roughly 64 patients are needed in each group.

With 90% power, we cannot use our rule of thumb.

$$\text{Recall that } n = \frac{2(z_{1-\alpha/2} + z_{1-\beta})^2}{(\delta/\sigma)^2}.$$

$z_1 - 0.05/2 = 1.96$ (see Table A.1); $z_{1-\beta} = z_{0.9} = 1.28$.

$$\text{Therefore, } n = \frac{2(1.96 + 1.28)^2}{(1/2)^2} = 84 \text{ (approximately)}.$$

Therefore, roughly 20 more patients are required with 90% power as opposed to 80% power.

5. The maximum power of a study is achieved when the proportions of subjects assigned to each group are equal. We have 80 recruits. Maximum power, therefore, is achieved with a sample size of 40 for each group.

Recall that $n = \dfrac{2(z_{1-\alpha/2} + z_{1-\beta})^2}{(\delta/\sigma)^2}$. Substituting the information we know into the aforementioned formula, we obtain

$$40 = \frac{2(1.96 + z_{1-\beta})^2}{(20/25)^2}.$$

Solving for $z_{1-\beta}$, we obtain $z_{1-\beta} = 1.62$.

This value of $z_{1-\beta}$ corresponds to a $1 - \beta$ of 0.9474 or power of 94.74%.

6. There are many permutations of blocks of six with two different treatment groups, e.g., ABAABA, BBAAAB, etc. The question is asking what the maximum imbalance could potentially be if at some point recruitment stops. Complete blocks of six are always balanced. The maximum imbalance would occur if the first three patients were assigned to the same treatment and then recruitment stopped:

i.e., AAA   stop

or BBB   stop

Either of the two aforementioned situations would lead to one group having three more subjects assigned to one treatment than the other. The maximum possible difference in size of groups is therefore 3. With blocks of size n, the maximum possible difference in size is always $n/2$.

References

1. Hulley SB, Cummings SR. *Designing Clinical Research: An Epidemiologic Approach.* Baltimore, Williams & Wilkins; 1988, p. 14.
2. Sackett DL, Richardson WS, Rosenberg W, Hayes, RB. *Evidence-Based Medicine: How to Practice & Teach EBM.* New York, Churchill Livingstone; 1997, pp 21–28.

Understanding the Results of Studies of Therapies

O B J E C T I V E S

1. Describe the idea and purpose of intention-to-treat analysis.
2. Define relative risk reduction (RRR) and calculate its value given the control and experimental event rates from a clinical trial.
3. Provide an example of how the RRR can be misleading.
4. Define absolute risk reduction, number needed to treat, and number needed to harm.
5. Define conditional probability.
6. Precisely define p value and describe the p-value fallacy.
7. List three important limitations of p values.
8. Describe how one form of Bayes theorem can be used to illustrate that a statistically significant p value often provides less evidence against the null hypothesis than is commonly believed.
9. Explain how a general formula of t test can be used to derive a formula for a 95% confidence interval (CI) for the difference in two means of continuously distributed data, when the underlying populations are normally distributed.
10. Describe the advantages of using CI instead of p values.
11. Describe how the degree of confidence for a CI (e.g., 90% versus 95%) and sample size influence its width.
12. Describe how CI can be used to accept or reject the null hypothesis.

5.1 Introduction

The content of this book is designed to help you make wise medical decisions. Often those decisions are based upon studies of new therapies. Indeed, analyzing the results of studies of therapies and then applying this analysis to the care of patients is among the most common and important tasks of physicians in clinical practice. This chapter is designed to help you interpret such results accurately and efficiently.

5.2 Intention-to-Treat

CASE 5.1

Your friend Danielle has recently completed a study comparing ginger root to placebo in the treatment of cold symptoms. The outcome is "number of days until complete resolution of cold symptoms." Fifty patients with the onset of cold symptoms within 24 hours are randomly assigned to ginger root initially, while 50 other patients are randomly assigned to placebo. All patients are asked to take three doses of each treatment daily until symptoms completely resolve. Unfortunately, 30 of the patients assigned to the ginger root group either did not take three doses a day or stopped taking the treatment prior to resolution of symptoms. By contrast, only five patients in the placebo did not take the treatment as prescribed. Should Danielle include the 30 patients who did not take ginger root as prescribed and the five patients who did not take placebo as prescribed in her final statistical analysis? Some of the patients assigned to the ginger root group did not take any ginger root at all. Should they be placed in the placebo group at the end of the trial for the purpose of analysis?

The correct answers to the questions in Case 5.1 are based upon a now widely accepted principle in the analysis of clinical trials known as *intention-to-treat*. In simple terms, the principle of intention-to-treat can be described as the following:

Once subjects are randomized to a particular group, they must remain in that group for analysis.

Essentially, intention-to-treat means "analyze as randomized." For Danielle's study, for example, the 30 patients assigned to the ginger root group who did not comply with treatment should be included in the ginger root group at the end of the study for analysis, regardless of whether they missed any or all pills or dropped out of the study altogether. At first, intention-to-treat might not seem rational. Would you not want to include only people who had taken the treatment correctly in the treatment group to determine the true effect of ginger root? There are several important reasons why intention-to-treat is the correct guiding principle for analysis of results. First, by keeping subjects in their assigned group regardless of circumstances, we are more closely simulating the "real life" situation. After all, in real life many patients do not take medications as prescribed. For example, the effectiveness of contraceptives (e.g., birth control pills) is described in two ways. There is the "method failure rate" which means that if the contraceptive is used correctly all the time, it will result in a certain number of accidental pregnancies. There is also the "user failure rate" which reflects the rate of failure among typical women who use the contraceptive. The user failure rate for contraceptives is generally higher than the method failure rate. It more accurately reflects the real-life situation.

The second very important reason for intention-to-treat analysis is because it *preserves the value of randomization*. As discussed in Chapter 4, the primary purpose of randomization is to distribute confounders evenly between groups so that two groups are as similar as possible at the outset of a study. Let us say that we decided not to include the 30 patients who did not comply fully with ginger root therapy in the analysis of Danielle's study. At the outset of the study, Danielle had two very similar groups. At the end of the study, one group is missing people who were unable or unwilling to comply with one of the treatments. It is possible that the subjects who did not comply fully with treatment differ systematically in some way from those who do. For example, perhaps those who did not comply had cold symptoms that were less severe than those who did. Randomization was used to create two roughly equal groups. By excluding the noncompliant subjects from the ginger root group, we are left with two groups that are no longer equal because a confounding variable may be responsible for noncompliance. The internal validity of our results would be compromised.

Intention-to-treat has become an important standard part of the evaluation of studies of therapies. Articles about new therapies will routinely indicate whether analysis was according to intention-to-treat. Let us assume that intention-to-treat was used for the Ceprotex study discussed in Chapter 4 and examine the results.

5.3 Results of Ceprotex Study

Assume that the Ceprotex study was completed successfully. The results are presented in Table 5.1. We will dissect each of these as we proceed through the chapter.

The table lists two events (stroke and GI bleeding). Let us begin by looking at the incidence of stroke. A quick calculation reveals that Ceprotex appears to prevent more strokes. Out of 322 patients, 24 or roughly 7.5% patients who received Ceprotex had a stroke compared to 47/317 or roughly 14.8% of patients who received coumadin. These proportions are known as *event rates*. The event rate corresponding to the new treatment

TABLE 5.1   Ceprotex vs. Coumadin in Prevention of Stroke

	Ceprotex ($n = 322$)	Coumadin ($n = 317$)	p Value
5-Year Stroke Incidence	24	47	0.015
Gastrointestinal Bleeding	12	7	0.04

under study is known as the *experimental event rate* (EER). The event rate corresponding to the new treatment is compared to what is known as the *control event rate* (CER). We can quantify the difference in event rates in different ways. One common measure is the *relative risk reduction* (RRR).

$$\text{RRR} = \frac{\text{CER} - \text{EER}}{\text{CER}}.$$

The RRR is the difference in event rates as a proportion of the CER. In our case,

$$\text{RRR} = \frac{47/317 - 24/322}{47/317} = \text{approximately } 0.50 \text{ (or } 50\% \text{)}.$$

This RRR can be interpreted in the following way:

Compared to coumadin, Ceprotex is associated with a 50% RRR in the 5-year incidence of stroke.

This sounds impressive, and within the context of this study, it is impressive. Sometimes, however, the RRR can be misleading because it fails to discriminate large treatment effects from small ones. Consider two separate studies of two therapies A and B (control). In the first study, 7% of patients who received therapy A died versus 77% who received therapy B. Therefore,

$$\text{RRR} = \frac{0.77 - 0.07}{0.77} = 0.91 \text{ (or } 91\% \text{)}.$$

In the second study, 0.07% of patients who received therapy A died versus 0.77% who received therapy B. Therefore,

$$\text{RRR} = \frac{0.0077 - 0.0007}{0.0077} = 0.91 \text{ (or } 91\% \text{)}.$$

In the first study, the majority of patients who received treatment B are dying. In the second study, deaths are very uncommon in both treatment groups. Despite this, the two studies reveal the same RRR. Relatively small differences in event rates can be exaggerated when only the RRR is used to describe the results of therapies. Companies or individuals wishing to promote specific products as superior to others often use the RRR for this purpose. For this reason, a different measure of effect based on event rates is needed.

The *absolute risk reduction* (ARR) is simply the absolute difference in event rates. For our Ceprotex study,

$$\text{ARR} = 47/317 - 24/322 = 0.074.$$

The ARR can be interpreted in the following way:

If 100 people were treated with Ceprotex and 100 people were treated with coumadin, 7.4 fewer people in the Ceprotex group would suffer a stroke over a 5-year period.

This interpretation of the ARR sounds awkward. We could make it seem more rational by saying that approximately 7 fewer people in the Ceprotex group would suffer a stroke. The ARR is not usually used directly but rather to obtain a more valuable statistic. If 100 patients with atrial fibrillation need to be treated with Ceprotex to prevent 7.4 strokes, how many people need to be treated to prevent one stroke? A little algebra is all that is needed:

$$\frac{100 \text{ patients}}{7.4 \text{ strokes prevented}} = \frac{X \text{ number of patients}}{1.0 \text{ stroke prevented}}.$$

$$X = 100/7.4 = 13.5 \text{ (or approximately 14).}$$

Approximately 14 people need to be treated with Ceprotex compared to coumadin to prevent one stroke. This number is commonly used to report the clinical significance of studies of therapies and is known as the *number needed to treat* (NNT). NNT can be expressed as

$$NNT = 1/ARR.$$

This NNT is defined as the number of people who need to be treated with one therapy compared to another to prevent one adverse event. NNT is a valuable measure of the usefulness of a new therapy. If the NNT is very high, meaning that many people need to be treated to prevent one adverse outcome, the new therapy may not be worth adopting into clinical practice. How high is too high? This is a difficult question to answer. It depends very much on the severity of the disease being treated, the costs of the new therapy, the therapy's adverse effects, etc. Numbers needed to treat for therapies that have been adopted into practice, as you might expect, are quite variable. Only 1.1 patients need to be treated with a combination of drugs to eradicate *Helicobacter pylori* (versus placebo), the bacteria responsible for many stomach and duodenal ulcers. Approximately 16 patients need to be treated with antibiotics (versus placebo) after a dog bite to prevent one infection. Twenty patients with heart attacks need to be treated with a combination of the drugs streptokinase and aspirin to prevent one death within 5 weeks.

Let us now consider the outcome of GI bleeding. Out of 322 patients who took Ceprotex 12 (3.7%) suffered this outcome compared with just 7 out of 317 (2.2%) patients who took coumadin. In this case, Ceprotex confers a disadvantage. The difference between these two rates is

$0.037 - 0.022 = 0.015$. This is an absolute risk *increase* of 0.015 of GI bleeding with Ceprotex. Taking the inverse of this number we obtain approximately 67. This number is known as the *number needed to harm* (NNH). It is interpreted in the following way:

If 67 people are treated with Ceprotex instead of coumadin, 1 extra person will suffer GI bleeding.

We now have two measures, the NNT and NNH, which can be used to translate event rates into statistics that are more meaningful for the care of patients. Both statistics offer a valuable perspective upon the usefulness of new therapies. An NNT of 100, for example, for a new treatment for a benign condition (such as tension headaches) means that if 100 extra people are treated with the new treatment instead of an older one, one extra headache would be cured. Most people would find adopting such a treatment unacceptable.

5.4 Interpretation of the *p* Value

Table 5.2 includes *p values*. The meaning of the *p* value should be clear when you consider the tests of significance we discussed in Chapter 2 and the way in which studies of therapies are designed as discussed in Chapter 4. Recall that in designing studies, we begin with the assumption of the null hypothesis, then carry out the study and perform tests of significance to see if the results are consistent with the null hypothesis. If the probability of obtaining those results under the assumption of the null hypothesis is below a prespecified level of significance (usually α of less than 0.05), then we reject the null hypothesis and conclude that the treatments being compared are not equivalent. The *p* value is simply the probability of obtaining a result under the assumption of the null hypothesis. When we designed our Ceprotex study, we set $\alpha = 0.05$. The *p* value for 5-year incidence of stroke is 0.015. We should reject the null hypothesis and conclude that Ceprotex and coumadin are not equivalent. The result that Ceprotex is different from coumadin is said to be *statistically significant*.

Unfortunately, *p* values are frequently misinterpreted by physicians. Mathematically, the meaning of the *p* value can be expressed using the idea of *conditional probability*. Conditional probability is simply the probability of an event given that a previous event has already occurred. In Chapter 3, we discussed Bayes theorem and the idea of a newborn calculating the probability of the sun rising each day given that the sun rose the previous day. This is a conditional probability. Algebraically, the conditional probability of an event B, given that an event A has already occurred is given by

$$p\,(B|A).$$

TABLE 5.2   Relation between Fixed Sample Size p Values and Minimun Bayes Factors and the Effect of Such Evidence on the Probability of the Null Hypothesis

p Value (z Score)	Minimum Bayes Factor	Decrease in Probability of the Null Hypothesis (%)		Strength of Evidence
		From	To No Less Than	
0.10	**0.26**	75	44	Weak
(1.64)	(1/3.8)	50	21	
		17	5	
0.05	**0.15**	75	31	Moderate
(1.96)	(1/6.8)	50	13	
		26	5	
0.03	**0.095**	75	22	Moderate
(2.17)	(1/11)	50	9	
		33	5	
0.01	**0.036**	75	10	Moderate to Strong
(2.58)	(1/28)	50	3.5	
		60	5	
0.001	**0.005**	75	1	Strong to very strong
(3.28)	(1/216)	50	0.5	
		92	5	

Reproduced with permission from Goodman SN. Toward evidence-based medical statistics. 2: The Bayes factor. Ann Intern Med 1999;130:1008.

The vertical line, "|" is read "conditional upon." When we perform tests of significance for studies of therapies we assume that the null hypothesis is true (i.e., the null hypothesis has already occurred). The p value can therefore be expressed as

$$p \text{ value} = p \text{ (results}|H_{o})$$

In words, this conditional probability is *the probability of getting the results assuming the null hypothesis is true* or, *the probability of getting the results assuming there is no difference between the treatments.* Often p values are misinterpreted because this definition is intuitively difficult to understand. Physicians are usually less interested in the probability of getting the results assuming there is no difference and more interested in the probability of there being no difference given the results. The probability of no difference given the results seems easier and a more logical basis upon which to draw conclusions about studies of therapy. The p value is frequently interpreted incorrectly as

$$p \text{ value} = p\,(H_o|\text{results})\,(\textit{incorrect!}).$$

This common misinterpretation is known as the *p-value fallacy*.[1] It is not possible through the methods we discussed in Chapter 4 to calculate the probability of the null hypothesis conditional upon the results, because we started with the assumption that the null hypothesis is true.

CASE 5.2

Your friend Charles has just completed a trial of two therapies for viral meningitis, A and B. The outcome was number of days until cure and was a mean of 7.3 days for treatment A and 9.9 days for treatment B. A *t* test was used to compare the two means. The *p* value obtained was 0.04. Charles concluded that based on the results of the study, there was only a 4% chance of there being no difference between the two treatments. Very confident that the two treatments are not equivalent, Charles has stopped treating patients with B completely. How is Charles' interpretation incorrect and what are its consequences?

Charles has subscribed to the *p*-value fallacy. Assuming the null hypothesis is true, there is a 4% chance of obtaining the difference in means he observed or a greater difference in the trial. This is not the same thing as there being a 4% chance of no difference in the two treatments. Does the *p*-value fallacy matter? Some argue that physicians and others have been misinterpreting the meaning of the *p* value for years without adverse consequences. Accurate interpretation is important, however, because small *p* values are actually less significant than many physicians believe them to be. Physicians want to know the probability of the null hypothesis. Dr. Stephen Goodman has described a way to illuminate the true significance of the *p* value using information about the probability of the null hypothesis in one form of Bayes theorem[2]:

$$\text{Prior odds of null hypothesis} \times \text{Bayes factor} = \text{Posterior odds of null hypothesis.}$$

Notice the similarities of this form of Bayes theorem to the form we discussed in Chapter 3 for diagnostic tests. The prior odds of the null hypothesis, like the *pretest odds of disease* is subjective. The Bayes factor is equivalent to the likelihood ratio for diagnostic tests and is defined as

$$\frac{p\,(\text{Results}|H_o)}{p\,(\text{Results}|H_1)}.$$

H_1 represents an alternative hypothesis, e.g., one treatment is 10% better than another. Consider the following example. You are about to compare two treatments, X and Y. Based on prior studies and general experience with the two drugs, you decide that there is a 50% chance that the two therapies are equivalent. The prior odds of the null hypothesis, therefore, are

$$\text{Odds} = 0.5/1 - 0.5 = 1:1.$$

Upon completion of the study, you obtain a difference in the means of the two treatments of "10" (A superior to B). The corresponding *p* value is 0.04. The alternative hypothesis that is most likely is the one *based on the results we observed*. In other words, the hypothesis "A is associated with a mean treatment effect 10 greater than B" is the alternative hypothesis that is most likely. Though this hypothesis is more likely than any other, the results also provide some support to other alternative hypotheses (e.g., a difference in means of 15, 20, etc.). This is one of the fundamental differences between this *Bayesian* approach to the interpretation of results of studies of therapy and a simple approach based only on the *p* value. In the simple *p* value approach, we are only concerned with whether the results are consistent with the null hypothesis or not. With a Bayesian approach, we are concerned with *which hypotheses are most likely* given the results. The actual calculation of the *p* [results|H_1] is complicated. (Please see Annotated Bibliography for references that describe the details.) For the sake of simplicity, let us assume for our example that *p*[result of 10| A is 10 better than B] is 0.28, or 7 times greater than *p*[result of 10|H_o], which is our *p* value of 0.04. We now have a Bayes factor of

$$\frac{p\,(\text{Results}|H_o)}{p\,(\text{Results}|H_1)} = \frac{0.04}{0.28} = \frac{1}{7}.$$

Our posterior odds of the null hypothesis are therefore given by

$$1/1 \times 1/7 = 1/7.$$

A *p* value of 0.04 looks very significant. In this hypothetical situation, however, after the results of the study are obtained, the null hypothesis still has one-seventh as much support as the most likely alternative hypothesis. The numbers selected for this example may be arbitrary, but Goodman describes a precise "exchange rate" for *p* values and "minimum Bayes factors" (the smallest value of the Bayes factor, i.e., the one that uses the most likely alternative hypothesis). *p* Values, their corresponding Bayes factors, and their impact upon the probability of the null hypothesis are given in Table 5.2.

The strength of evidence refers to evidence against the null hypothesis. A *p* value of 0.05, for example, translates to a minimum Bayes factor of 0.15.

If we decide that the prior probability of the null hypothesis is 50% (i.e., odds of 1 to 1), the posterior probability of the null hypothesis remains 13%. This is certainly much higher than 5%, which is what many would misinterpret the probability of the null hypothesis to be. In fact, our prior probability of the null hypothesis would have to be a mere 26% (i.e., we are very optimistic about two treatments being different), before the p value and true $p[H_o|results]$ are equivalent.

This form of Bayes theorem is somewhat esoteric. For your purposes, it is useful to help you understand that small p values are not as significant as they might first appear. In the interpretation of studies of therapies, it is more important for you to accurately interpret the p value instead of using this alternative method of interpretation using Bayes thereom.

5.5 Limitations of p Values

The preceding discussion describes an important limitation of p values: the ease with which they are misinterpreted. They have two important additional limitations. First, p values tell us only if an observed difference between treatments is statistically significant. They do not provide information about the magnitude of the difference. Let us say, for example, that a difference between two mean treatment effects is 1.6 and the p value for this difference is 0.04. If the study was designed with α of 0.05, we would describe the difference as statistically significant. What is unclear is how closely the observed difference approximates the true difference in the population. Is the true difference exactly 1.6, or does the true difference lie in a range around 1.6, say between 1.2 and 2.0? The importance of this limitation will become more apparent in the next section.

Another important limitation of p values is that very small p values can result not from dramatic differences between the treatments being compared, but from large sample sizes. For example, recall the formula for the t test from Chapter 2:

$$t = \frac{\overline{O} - \overline{U}}{\sqrt{s^2/n_{\overline{O}} + s^2/n_{\overline{U}}}}$$

Notice that the value of t is directly proportional to the observed difference in the means of the outcome between the two groups being compared and directly proportional to the square root of the sample sizes of each of the samples. This means that smaller observed differences in means can be compensated for by larger samples to generate the same value of t. Furthermore, if you take a close look at the table of critical values of t in the Appendix (Table A.3), you will notice that smaller values of t are needed to reach the same critical value (e.g., 0.05) as the number of degrees of freedom increases. As noted, the number of degrees of freedom v is equal to

$n_{\overline{O}} + n_{\overline{U}} - 2$. Even small differences, therefore, can be associated with small p values and be statistically significant if the sample size is large enough. Such small differences between two treatments may not have clinical significance.

5.6 Confidence Intervals: A Better Alternative

CASE 5.3

Your friend Marlene has recently completed a study comparing two treatments for migraine headaches, A and B. The primary outcome is "number of hours to complete relief of symptoms." The mean for treatment A is 4.2 hours, while the mean for treatment B is 5 hours. The standard error of this difference in means is 0.3 hours. There are 30 subjects in each group being compared. How can the statistical significance of this study be expressed? Assume that the outcome in the population being studied is normally distributed.

A t test should be used to test the difference between the two means. Recall that

$$t = \frac{\text{difference of sample means}}{\text{standard error of difference in sample means}}.$$

For Case 5.2, $t = 0.8/0.3 = 2.4$; there are $30 + 30 - 2$ or 58 degrees of freedom. Looking at the critical values of t in Table A.3 (two-tailed) for 58 degrees of freedom, you will find a value of 2.002 at a level of significance of 0.05. In fact, our value of t is close to the value for the level of significance of 0.02. Treatment A is therefore statistically different from treatment B. We can report this as $p < 0.05$ or $p = 0.02$ (approximately), bearing in mind all the limitations of p values we have just discussed.

Now let us explore an alternative to this method of rejecting or accepting the null hypothesis based on p values. In fact, forget about the null hypothesis for a moment. We use samples to estimate the true differences in the populations from which they were drawn. The aforementioned definition of t is based on the idea that there are no differences between the treatments being compared (i.e., null hypothesis). Alternatively, we can define t as[3]

$$t = \frac{\text{difference of sample means} - \text{actual difference in population means}}{\text{standard error of difference in sample means}}.$$

Algebraically, this becomes

$$t = \frac{(\overline{X}_1 - \overline{X}_2) - (\mu_1 - \mu_2)}{s_{\overline{X}_1 - \overline{X}_2}}.$$

Note that if there is no difference in populations, meaning the two samples are drawn from the same population, $\mu_1 - \mu_2$ becomes 0 and our equation for t becomes the same as it was under the null hypothesis. *The aforementioned equation, therefore, is a more general form of t that takes into consideration not only the case when the null hypothesis is true but also when it is not true and there is a true difference between the population means, represented by $\mu_1 - \mu_2$.*

The statistic t is normally distributed, which means that its curve has a symmetric shape and individual values of t can be defined by percentiles. The threshold value of t we are usually concerned with is the value that defines the most extreme 5% of values. This value of t is the same as that which corresponds to our level of significance or type 1 error rate (α) of 0.05. In general, when using a two-tailed t test, we are concerned with two threshold values: t_α and $-t_\alpha$.

If we repeat our study using two different samples each time, 100 $(1 - \alpha)$ percent of the time, the value of t will fall between t_α and $-t_\alpha$. In other words,

$$-t_\alpha < \frac{(\overline{X}_1 - \overline{X}_2) - (\mu_1 - \mu_2)}{s_{\overline{X}_1 - \overline{X}_2}} < t_\alpha.$$

Rearranging this equation algebraically, we obtain

$$(\overline{X}_1 - \overline{X}_2) - t_\alpha s_{\overline{X}_1 - \overline{X}_2} < \mu_1 - \mu_2 < (\overline{X}_1 - \overline{X}_2) + t_\alpha s_{\overline{X}_1 - \overline{X}_2}.$$

Notice that the true difference between the two populations means now lies in an interval whose size depends upon the difference between the sample means, the level of significance and its corresponding value of t, and the standard error of the difference in the sample means. The difference thus defined is known as a *confidence interval* (CI) for the difference in means. The most common value used for α is 0.05. The interval we are usually concerned with is therefore

$$(\overline{X}_1 - \overline{X}_2) - t_{0.05} s_{\overline{X}_1 - \overline{X}_2} < \mu_1 - \mu_2 < (\overline{X}_1 - \overline{X}_2) + t_{0.05} s_{\overline{X}_1 - \overline{X}_2}.$$

This is the *95% CI*. If Marlene repeated her study 100 times, the true difference in means would lie in this interval 95 times and outside of it 5 times. The interval therefore provides a measure of the precision of her estimate of the difference in means based on her single study. We can say that we are *confident* that based on her single study, the true difference in means will lie in this interval 95 times if the study were repeated 100 times. Let us now calculate this interval. We know that the difference in sample means is 0.8 and the standard error of this difference is 0.3. The value of t corresponding to α of 0.05 and 58 degrees of freedom is approximately 2.

Our interval becomes

$$0.8 - 2 \times 0.3 < \mu_1 - \mu_2 < 0.8 + 2 \times 0.3$$

Or,

$$0.2 < \mu_1 - \mu_2 < 1.4.$$

Based on her single study, the true difference in means will lie between 0.2 and 1.4 95% of the time. The information is usually abbreviated in the form

$$95\% \text{ CI } (0.2, 1.4).$$

Remember that the CI is a measure of the precision of our estimate of the difference based on the results of the study. This estimate is 0.8 and its 95% CI is usually placed next to it. We can summarize the study in the form

$$\text{Difference} = 0.8, 95\% \text{ CI } (0.2, 1.4).$$

You will encounter this form frequently in the medical literature. Unlike the method of rejecting or accepting the null hypothesis based upon the p value, which tells us only if a difference is statistically significant or not, CI provide a measure of the *magnitude* of the difference. In Case 5.2, for example, we know that the difference in treatments could be as low as 0.2 or as high as 1.4. The width of a CI (the difference between the two values which define it) is a measure of the *precision* of our estimate of the difference. A very wide CI for an estimate tells us that there is a great deal of uncertainty about the estimate.

5.7 Principles of Interpretation of CI

Section 5.6 described where CI for the difference between two means come from when the underlying populations are assumed to be normal. Chapter 2 included a number of statistical tests. Both p values and CI can be calculated for the results of these and other statistical tests and other types of statistics as well. It is possible, for example, to calculate 95% CI for individual likelihood ratios that describe the precision and magnitude of the likelihood ratio derived from a diagnostic study. You might encounter something like the following in a diagnostic paper:

$$\text{LR}_{(+)} = 6.5, 95\% \text{ CI } (3.5, 9.5).$$

Overall, CI are more versatile than p values and have found an increasingly larger number of applications in which they describe magnitude and precision. Some basic principles of interpretation apply to all CI:

1. For the same study, the 90% CI for an estimate is *narrower* than the 95% CI. For example, for Marlene's study, the 95% CI is 0.2–1.4. The 90% CI could be something like 0.4–1.2. Intuitively this makes sense. We can be 95% sure that a true value lies within a broad range. We are less sure (i.e., 90% in this case) that the true value lies within a smaller range. Consider the following example. A group of 100 average men are assembled in a room. Knowing nothing about them, how sure are you that the mean height of the men lies between 3'11" and 7'11" ? Hopefully, you are 100% or close to 100% sure, since this is a very broad range of adult-male heights. How sure are you that the mean height lies between 5'9" and 5'11" ? You are probably much less sure. Similarly, the higher the percent confidence for the same study, the wider the interval.

2. Larger sample sizes yield narrower CI. This also makes sense intuitively. The larger the sample size we use, the more our sample approximates the underlying population. We would therefore be more sure of our estimates.

3. CI, like p values, can be used to accept or reject the null hypothesis. If the CI includes a value that describes no difference between two treatments (usually 0, but sometimes a ratio of 1:1), then there is no statistical difference between the two treatments and the null hypothesis should be accepted. Consider the following interval:

Difference in effects = 81.3, 95% CI $(-30, 132.6)$

The CI is wide and includes the number zero. This means that if the study was repeated many times, the true difference would lie in this broad interval, which *includes zero* 95% of the time. Under these circumstances, we should accept the null hypothesis. Note that if the CI describes no difference, then the corresponding p value must also describe no difference (in this case p must be > 0.05). "No difference" between two treatments can be described as an absolute difference of zero as it is above, but is more often expressed as the ratio of the effect of one treatment to another of 1:1. We will discuss such ratios later in the book.

PROBLEMS

1. The results of a trial of a new antibiotic for community-acquired pneumonia are shown in Table 5.3. The new antibiotic (NewBot) was

TABLE 5.3   Event Rates Among Patients with Community-Acquired Pneumonia

Event	NewBot (n = 100)	Azithromycin (n = 100)	p Value
Cure after 1 week	74	61	0.003
Hospitalization	12	15	0.004
Death	2	3	0.002
Diarrhea	40	25	0.005

compared to azithromycin, an older, widely used antibiotic (control) with respect to certain key outcomes.

Calculate the CER, EER, and RRR of *not* being cured, being hospitalized, or dying from pneumonia based on the information given in Table 5.3. Calculate the ARR, NNT for the three outcomes, and the NNH for the outcome of diarrhea.

2. The mean number of days until cure was 6.2 days in the NewBot group and 7 days in the azithromycin group. The standard deviation of number of days until cure for community-acquired pneumonia is approximately 2.4 days. The outcome of number of days until cure is always normally distributed. Calculate the *p* value and 95% CI for the difference in the two mean days until cure.

3. Erin has recently completed a study to compare two different antibiotics, amoxicillin and erythromycin, for acute otitis media in children under the age of 24 months. Her principal outcome is the number of days until cure. She began the study believing that there is approximately a 50% chance that there is no difference between the two treatments with respect to this outcome. Upon completion of the study, she uses a *t* test to compare the mean number of days until cure between the two groups. Erythromycin was associated with a mean of 1.3 fewer days until cure than amoxicillin. The *p* value for this difference was 0.03. Nevertheless, Erin remains somewhat skeptical about using erythromycin instead of amoxicillin in all cases of acute otitis media in children under 24 months. Explain how Bayes theorem provides a reason for her skepticism.

SOLUTIONS TO PROBLEMS

1. If 74 and 61 people out of 100 are cured in the NewBot and azithromycin groups, respectively, then 26 and 39 people out of 100, respectively, are *not* cured. Calculations for event rates, RRR, ARR, NNT, and NNH are shown as follows:

I. CER (no cure) = 39/100 (39%).
EER (no cure) = 26/100 (26%).
RRR = (0.39 – 0.26)/0.39 = 0.33 (33%).

II. CER (hospitalization) = 15/100 (15%).
EER (hospitalization) = 12/100 (12%).
RRR = (0.15 – 0.12)/0.15 = 0.2 (20%).

III. CER (dying) = 3/100 (3%).
EER (dying) = 2/100 (2%).
RRR = (0.03 – 0.02)/0.03 = 0.33 (33%).

ARR (no cure) = 0.39 – 0.26 = 0.13; NNT = 1/ARR = 1/0.13 = 7.7 (roughly 8). Roughly eight people need to be treated with NewBot instead of azithromycin for one extra cure.

ARR (hospitalization) = 0.15 – 0.12 = 0.03; NNT = 1/ARR = 1/0.03 = 33.3 (roughly 33). Roughly 33 people need to be treated with New-Bot instead of azithromycin to prevent one hospitalization.

ARR (death) = 0.03 – 0.02 = 0.01; NNT = 1/ARR = 1/0.01 = 100. One-hundred people need to be treated with NewBot instead of azithromycin to prevent one death.

AR (increase) (diarrhea) = 0.4 – 0.25 = 0.15; NNH = 1/AR (increase) = 6.7 (roughly 7). If seven people are treated with NewBot instead of azithromycin, one extra person will suffer diarrhea.

2. Recall that t is defined as $t = \dfrac{\overline{O} - \overline{U}}{\sqrt{s^2/n_{\overline{O}} + s^2/n_{\overline{U}}}}$.

For this problem, this becomes

$$t = \frac{0.8}{\sqrt{2.4^2/100 + 2.4^2/100}} = 2.36.$$

We have 198 degrees of freedom. Our value of t occurs with a p of approximately 0.02 (p is therefore approximately 0.02). To calculate the 95% CI, we need $t_{0.05}$ and the denominator of our aforementioned equation for t.

For approximately 198 degrees of freedom, $t_{0.05}$ is roughly 1.97. The denominator in the equation for t (standard error of difference in means) is 0.34. Our 95% CI can be defined as

0.8 – 1.97(0.34) to 0.8 + 1.97(0.34), or 0.13 to 1.47.

The result can be summarized as difference = 0.8 days, 95% CI (0.13, 1.47).

Notice that the range in the estimate of the true difference is quite wide. You could not appreciate this by summarizing the result with a p value.

3. The minimum Bayes factor associated with a p value of 0.03 is 0.095. Erin began her study with a healthy dose of skepticism. Her pretest odds of the null hypothesis are 1:1. The posttests odds of the null hypothesis are therefore, $1:1 \times 0.095 = 0.095:1$. This translates to a posttest probability of the null hypothesis of roughly 9%. Based on her prior odds of the null hypothesis and what she observed in the study, therefore, the null hypothesis still has a significant probability of being true. This is why she remains skeptical about any true difference between the two treatments.

References

1. Goodman SN. Toward evidence-based medical statistics. 1: The P value fallacy. *Ann Intern Med* 1999;130(12):995–1004.
2. Goodman SN. Toward evidence-based medical statistics. 2: The Bayes factor. *Ann Intern Med* 1999;130(12):1005–1013.
3. Glantz SA. *Primer of Biostatistics*, 5th ed. New York: McGraw-Hill; 2002, p. 201.

Etiology

6

1. Define etiology.
2. Define anamnesis.
3. Distinguish between cohort and case-control studies and describe the advantages and disadvantages of each in studying the etiology of disease.
4. Describe three types of bias to which case-control studies are prone.
5. Distinguish between descriptive and analytic cohort studies.
6. Distinguish between prospective and retrospective cohort studies.
7. Define inception cohort.
8. Define relative risk (RR) and calculate the RR from the results of a cohort study.
9. Define odds ratio (OR) and calculate the OR from the results of a cohort or case-control study.
10. Explain why RR should not be used to describe the results of a case-control study.
11. Distinguish between internal and external controls for a cohort study.
12. Define logarithm and natural logarithm and explain why natural logarithms are frequently used in biostatistics.
13. Calculate the 95% CI for RR given the results of a cohort study and the 95% CI for an OR given the results of a cohort or case-control study.

6.1 Introduction

The word *etiology* is derived from the Greek words *aitia*, meaning cause, and *logos*, meaning words or speech. Etiology can be defined alternatively as the "cause of disease" or the "philosophical study of causation." One can talk about the "etiology of lung cancer" which includes transformation of cells upon exposure to cigarettes. So far, we have explored the design and analysis of studies about diagnosis and therapies. These are the types of studies that have the greatest direct impact upon patient care. For example, to the average, busy, practicing physician, a new study that links low dairy (calcium) consumption to bone fractures in children may be interesting, but it may be hard for the physician to determine exactly how the information should be used. They may ask themselves questions such as the following:

- Does this study mean that increasing dairy consumption is a good way to prevent fractures?
- How exactly do I determine if a child consumes too little dairy?
- Should I recommend increasing dairy consumption to my families with children?
- What precisely should I tell them about how much dairy is required to prevent fractures?
- Even if I do recommend increased dairy consumption, will my patients actually follow my advice?

Unless precise answers to these and other related questions are available, studies about the etiology of disease are difficult to translate into recommendations for clinical practice. Nevertheless, knowing how such studies are designed and should be interpreted is very important. As you might imagine from the aforementioned example, a study that suggests a cause for a particular disease raises new questions that can be explored by the methodologies we have discussed in Chapters 3–5. The study linking low dairy consumption to fractures might lead to a study designed to develop a quick diagnostic questionnaire to diagnose low dairy consumption among children. It might lead to a randomized, controlled trial comparing calcium supplementation to placebo with the outcome of number of fractures recorded in each group. Studies of etiology, therefore, are often important precursors to studies of diagnosis or therapies. Keeping up to date with such studies raises awareness of future studies that have a more direct impact upon patient care.

Even though they do not have a large direct and immediate impact upon patient care, studies of etiology are of intense interest among the general public. Scarcely a day goes by without a news report linking some environmental hazard, chemical or human behavior to disease. Such information is generally presented to the public poorly. News reports are often inaccurate or unnecessarily alarmist. Misinterpretation of studies of etiology can even lead to unhealthy behaviors. When the first reports of the benefits of red wine consumption upon cardiovascular health emerged several years ago, for example, many of my patients used them as an excuse to justify their high levels of alcohol consumption. It is the duty of physicians to explain the significance of studies of etiology to their patients accurately and to place the importance of such studies in the context of their patients' overall health. A middle-aged man, for example, who smokes heavily, overeats and does no exercise should probably work on these problems first before deciding to increase his red wine consumption.

6.2 Designs for Studies of Etiology

The causes of symptoms or diseases can be investigated in many ways. Troublesome side effects of medications, for example, are often discovered during the course of studies of therapies that use the randomized, controlled trial design. In general, the causes of disease are investigated through two study designs with which you should become familiar. *Cohort studies* involve following study subjects over a period of time. *Case-control* studies include people with and without a particular condition and look backward at what may have caused it. Much of the remainder of this chapter is devoted to the procedures and analysis of these two study designs.

6.3 Cohort Studies

Cohort studies are usually carried out for one of two purposes. Patients can be followed over a period of time to measure the incidence of disease (*descriptive cohort studies*). It is possible, for example, to follow a group of smokers over a 20-year period and determine how many of them develop lung cancer. More relevant to this chapter is the use of cohort studies to determine the relationship between *risk factors* and one or more outcomes (*analytic cohort studies*). A risk factor is simply something that may increase the risk of disease. Cigarette smoking, for example, is a risk factor for lung cancer. Cohort studies may be *prospective* or *retrospective*. In prospective cohort studies, the investigator assembles a group of subjects or "cohort" and measures risk factors or "predictor variables" before the outcome or outcomes of interest have occurred. In retrospective studies, the investigator defines a group of subjects and first measures predictor variables even though the outcome or outcomes have already occurred. In both types of studies, the outcome status is unknown at the time the predictor variables are measured. Recruiting 1000 smokers and following them for 10 years to determine which patients develop lung cancer is a prospective design. Looking through the medical records of 1000 smokers that include 10 years of data to determine how many developed lung cancer in that period is a retrospective design.

CASE 6.1

Your friend Stan has noticed recently that several children in his practice who live near a petroleum refinery develop asthma at a young age. The refinery produces a great deal of pollution in the form of nitrogen oxide. He would like to study the problem to determine if there is a relationship between nitrogen oxide exposure and asthma. How should he go about it and how should he analyze the results?

Imagine the possibility of carrying out a randomized clinical trial to answer Stan's question. A randomized, controlled trial is essentially a cohort study in which the factors under study or *exposures* are under the control of the investigator. It is impossible, however, not to mention completely unethical, to expose one of two groups of recruited subjects to nitrogen oxide and monitor the subjects for asthma. A prospective cohort design is a good way to answer the question. One could recruit a group of children who lived in a community with a refinery (though not necessarily very near it) and follow them over the course of 5 or more years to determine how many develop asthma. A single group of this type in a cohort study, all of whose members have something in common, is known as an *inception cohort*. This type of study would reveal the incidence of asthma in children exposed to nitrogen oxide. It does not give us an idea of whether similar children who were not exposed to nitrogen oxide develop asthma at the same or a different rate. For this reason, it is preferable to include two groups—one of which serves as a control and consists of children who were not exposed to nitrogen oxide. In double cohort studies of this type, control groups can be drawn from the same inception cohort and are known as *internal controls*. Alternatively, control groups can be assembled separately from outside the inception cohort (*external controls*). Stan could recruit children all from a local school (inception cohort) and then assemble two similar groups, one of which consisted of children who lived near the refinery and the other which did not (internal controls). Stan could also recruit a group of children who lived near the refinery and a similar group of children who lived in another neighborhood (external controls). Which type of control is used is often a matter of convenience. Using internal controls is more likely to yield two groups that are similar except with respect to the factor under study.

Let us assume that Stan assembles two groups: one group of children who live near the refinery and the other group of children who do not. All children are free of asthma at the start of the study. He follows them over a 5-year period and then, through their medical records, determines how many develop asthma in that time. The results of such cohort studies can be summarized using the general form of a 2×2 table as shown in Table 6.1.

TABLE 6.1   Algebraic Contingency Table for Cohort Studies

		Outcome		
		Present	**Absent**	**Total**
Exposed	Yes	a	b	a + b
	No	c	d	c + d
Total		a + c	b + d	a + b + c + d

The incidence of the outcome among subjects "exposed" is given by

$$a/(a + b).$$

The incidence of the outcome among subjects not "exposed" is given by

$$c/(c + d).$$

The ratio of these two incidences is known as the *relative risk* (RR) or alternatively as the *risk ratio*:

$$RR = \frac{a/a + b}{c/c + d}.$$

Note that the RR is a simple ratio of two incidences or event rates. It is not the same thing as the RRR discussed in Chapter 5. The RR can be used to describe the outcomes of studies of therapy. In general, however, RRR should not be used to describe the outcomes of cohort studies. The *odds ratio* (OR), a more versatile measure of the outcomes of both cohort and case control studies, will be discussed later in the chapter.

Notice that we are dealing with categorical data. The outcomes of cohort studies are either disease + or disease −. All statistics based upon samples are estimates of population parameters and are imprecise to some degree. Now that you have learned about CIs, we can quantify the degree of precision of the RR. The derivation of the formula for the CI as shown next is somewhat complicated. The formula itself is the following:

Lower boundary of CI $= {}_e\ln(RR) - z_{1-\alpha/2} \times \sqrt{b/an_1 + d/cn_2}$.

Upper boundary of CI $= {}_e\ln(RR) + z_{1-\alpha/2} \times \sqrt{b/an_1 + d/cn_2}$.

The formula makes use of logarithms. It has probably been sometime since you have used them and a brief review here will help you understand the formulae for CIs for both RRs and ORs. A logarithm is the inverse function of an exponent. More precisely, if

$b^n = x$, then the logarithm is the function that gives n: $\log_b x = n$.

We say, "the log *base b* of x, is n." Consider the following example.

$2^3 = 8$. Therefore, $\log_2 8 = 3$. Whenever you see "log" without the base specified, it implies that base 10 is used. For example, $\log 100 = 2$, because $10^2 = 100$. The inverse of the logarithm function is exponentiation and vice versa. The formula for CIs includes a very special type of logarithm, designated *ln*. This is known as the "natural logarithm"—so named for reasons that are beyond the scope of this book. The natural logarithm is the logarithm with base e, where e is approximately 2.71828. e can be defined by an infinite number of digits, like Π, the ratio of the circumference of a circle to its radius. If $e^n = x$, then $\ln(x) = n$. Biostatistics makes generous use of natural logarithms because the natural logarithm of a statistic is sometimes more likely to follow a familiar distribution (e.g., normal distribution) than the statistic itself. For example, $\ln(RR)$ more closely approximates a normal distribution than RR itself. The natural logarithm of a statistic can be taken, compared to the normal distribution to draw conclusions, and then reversed by exponentiation. This is what is going on in the formulae for the CI of an RR.

The remaining elements of the formulae should be familiar. In Chapter 5, z scores for CIs were discussed. a, b, c, and d are the values of the cell in the 2 × 2 table from which RR is calculated. n_1 and n_2 are the sizes of the two groups being compared in the cohort study. Let us return to Case 6.1. Assume that Stan's results take the form as shown in Table 6.2.

Stan has compared 100 children with and without exposure to nitrogen oxide. The RR is given by

$$RR = \frac{28/(28+72)}{7/(7+93)} = 4.$$

The RR can be interpreted as the following: *Children exposed to nitrogen oxide have a four fold increased risk of developing asthma compared to children unexposed to nitrogen oxide.*

Let us assume we are interested in the 95% CI ($\alpha = 0.05$) for the RR. The lower and upper boundaries are given by

$$_e\ln(4) - 1.96 \times \sqrt{[72/28 \times 100 + 93/7 \times 100]} = 1.83.$$

And,

$$_e\ln(4) + 1.96 \times \sqrt{[72/28 \times 100 + 93/7 \times 100]} = 8.73.$$

TABLE 6.2   Stan's Results

		Outcome		
		Develops Asthma	No Asthma	Total
Exposed to nitrogen oxide	Yes	28	72	100
	No	7	93	100
Total		35	165	200

One could summarize Stan's results as: RR = 4, 95% CI (1.83, 8.73). Since this 95% CI does not include zero, one can conclude that the RR is statistically significant. By doing so we are *rejecting the null hypothesis* that there is no increased risk of asthma upon exposure to nitrogen oxide (i.e., the RR is 1).

6.4 Case-Control Studies

Cohort studies measure predictor variables, which can be risk factors for disease or exposures of any kind, and follow patients with these variables forward in time. The actual period of follow-up can be in the future (prospective cohort) or past (retrospective cohort). By contrast, case-control studies are almost always retrospective. First, subjects with and without a particular condition are identified. Subjects with the condition are known as *cases*, while those without it are known as *controls*. Next, investigators look back in time to see what predictor variables could explain why the cases got the condition and the controls did not. The outcomes of case-control studies provide a measure of the strength of association between a predictor variable and a disease.

Case-control studies have been appearing increasingly more often in the medical literature over the past 40 years. They are relatively simple to carry out and may suggest etiologies for diseases, knowledge of which may lead to the development of therapies or diagnostic procedures. Case-control studies themselves evolved out of an interest in cases in general. The idea that "a case of tuberculosis," for example, includes specific features is of course widely accepted today. Until the seventeenth century, however, defining diseases by characteristic signs, symptoms, and pathology was uncommon. Diseases were thought to be different responses to environmental factors. Lack of fresh air, for example, could manifest itself in many different ways (fever, cough, fatigue, etc.).

Once the idea of cases was accepted, people began to ask questions about etiology: why did people living in different circumstances all develop the same specific disease? Establishing etiology often involves the process of *anamnesis*—collecting information about the events in a patient's life that are thought to be relevant to the patient's disease through a formal interview.

CASE 6.2

Soft-tissue sarcoma is a very rare form of cancer. Your friend Pedro suspects that exposure to the herbicide 2,4-D is a cause. How should he go about investigating this possibility and analyzing the results?

One could assemble a group of individuals who just happen to be exposed to the herbicide and a comparable group who had not and then wait for the appearance of soft-tissue sarcoma among the recruited subjects. The impracticality of this approach should be obvious. It takes many years for cancer to develop. A prospective cohort design, therefore, would require following patients over a long period of time. This would be expensive and difficult, since many patients may drop out of the study. Furthermore, even if this were possible, the cancer is quite rare. If only a small number of subjects exposed to the herbicide were followed for a long time, none may develop the cancer. A useful prospective cohort study, therefore, would require following a very large number of patients to allow for the appearance of a sufficient number of cases of cancer upon which to draw conclusions. A case-control approach is more appropriate in this situation.

The first step is to select a sample of patients from the population of patients with soft tissue sarcoma. Since soft tissue sarcoma is a well-defined disease, this should be relatively straightforward. The challenge is in finding enough cases to make the results of the study meaningful. Let us say Pedro manages to recruit 100 patients with soft-tissue sarcoma into his study. The next step is to recruit a similar number of controls. Ideally, the controls would be identical to the cases in every way except that they do not have soft tissue sarcoma. It is important that Pedro is able to determine whether the controls were exposed to the herbicide to the same degree of accuracy as he is able to determine whether the cases were exposed. People with rare diseases such as soft tissue sarcoma are often more conscientious of potential etiologies and may be able to more accurately describe their exposures than people without such diseases. Anamnesis, therefore, is prone to inaccuracy. It may be possible to determine exposure more objectively such as through medical or occupational records. Let us say Pedro is able to recruit 100 patients similar in every way to the cases except that none have soft-tissue sarcoma (as you might expect, control patients are easier to recruit than patients with sarcoma). Through methodical interviews, he is able to ascertain whether any of the study recruits were exposed to 2,4-D. He obtains the results as shown in Table 6.3.

TABLE 6.3   Pedro's Results

		Outcome		
		Has Sarcoma	No Sarcoma	Total
Exposed to 2,4-D	Yes	12	3	15
	No	88	97	185
Total		100	100	200

Notice the similarity of this table of the results of a case-control study to that of the results of a cohort study. There are, however, important differences. In Case 6.1, the table reads: *develops* asthma. In the case-control study, the cases already have the disease. The table therefore reads: *has* sarcoma. How should these results be analyzed? It is tempting to use the RR as a summary. Intuitively, an important problem may have struck you. The RR describes the *risk* of developing a particular condition based on the presence of some predictor variable. In a case-control study, we cannot talk about the risk of developing a condition because subjects have been chosen on the basis of having or not having the condition. Let us put it another way: RRs are ratios of the incidences of diseases in two different samples. You cannot calculate the incidence of disease when you started by choosing patients with and without the disease. We need another measure of the strength of association between exposure to 2,4-D and soft-tissue sarcoma. Let us return to an algebraic version of a 2 × 2 table as given in Table 6.4. This one is for case-control studies.

In order to interpret the results of a case-control study, let us not talk about the risk of developing a condition among subjects exposed or unexposed, but rather the odds of exposure among the cases and the odds of exposure among the controls. This makes more sense than talking about the "risk of developing a disease" since we are starting with what we know (whether a subject has a disease or not) and then collecting information about exposure. The odds of exposure among cases (disease present) is simply the ratio a/c.

The odds of exposure among the controls (disease absent) is b/d.

The *OR* is defined as

$$\frac{a/c}{b/d}.$$

or

$$OR = ad/bc.$$

TABLE 6.4   Algebraic Table for Case-Control Studies

		Outcome		
		Disease Present	**Absent**	**Total**
Exposed	Yes	a	b	a + b
	No	c	d	c + d
Total		a + c	b + d	a + b + c + d

The OR is extremely versatile, and you will find it in many different types of studies including as an outcome measure of randomized, controlled trials. Although the RR cannot be used to summarize the results of case-control studies, the OR can be used to summarize the results of cohort studies. In cohort studies, however, we need to define the odds a little differently, since when we begin we do not know who has or does not have the disease. For a cohort study, consider the odds of *developing disease* among those who are exposed, which is

$$a/b.$$

Also consider the odds of *developing disease* among those not exposed:

$$c/d.$$

The OR is $\dfrac{a/b}{c/d} = \dfrac{ad}{bc}$.

Notice that the formula for the OR remains the same. It is the interpretation that is different for the two different kinds of studies. For a case-control study, the OR is *the odds of exposure among those with the disease compared to the odds of exposure among those without the disease.* For a cohort study, the OR is *the odds of disease among those exposed compared to the odds of disease among those unexposed.* For very rare disease outcomes in cohort studies, the OR approximates the RR. Recall the formula for RR:

$$RR = \frac{a/a+b}{c/c+d}.$$

If the disease outcome is rare, a is very small compared to b, and c is very small compared to d. Under such circumstances,

$$RR \approx \frac{a/b}{c/d} = OR.$$

Like RRs, ORs are based upon samples and are therefore inherently imprecise. It is therefore important to quantify the degree of imprecision with CIs:

Lower boundary of CI $= {}_e\ln(OR) - z_{1-\alpha/2} \times \sqrt{1/a + 1/b + 1/c + 1/d}.$

Upper boundary of CI $= {}_e\ln(OR) + z_{1-\alpha/2} \times \sqrt{1/a + 1/b + 1/c + 1/d}.$

In our algebraic 2 × 2 table (Table 6.4), a, b, c, and d are the values.

Let us return to Case 6.2. The OR in Pedro's study is

$$\frac{12 \times 97}{3 \times 88} = 4.41.$$

We would interpret this in the following way:

Among subjects with soft-tissue sarcoma compared to subjects without soft-tissue sarcoma, the odds of exposure to 2,4-D is approximately 4.4 to 1.

The higher the OR, the stronger is the association between the exposure and the disease. The 95% CI for Pedro's OR is given by

$$_e\ln(4.41) - 1.96 \times \sqrt{1/12 + 1/3 + 1/88 + 1/97} = 1.20$$

and

$$_e\ln(4.41) + 1.96 \times \sqrt{1/12 + 1/3 + 1/88 + 1/97} = 16.1.$$

The results of Pedro's study can therefore be summarized with OR = 4.41, 95% CI (1.20, 16.1). This is a very wide CI, but note that it does not include 1.0. Like a CI for an absolute difference in two means that includes zero, a CI for an OR that includes 1 means that the results are not statistically significant. For Pedro's study we would reject the null hypothesis and say the results are statistically significant.

6.5 Cohort Versus Case-Control Studies

Both cohort and case-control designs are important tools in a researcher's arsenal. Each has distinct advantages and disadvantages. Cohort studies, unlike case-control studies, can more reliably establish a sequence of events. Following children exposed to lead forward in time to see which ones develop hyperactivity disorder, for example, begins by establishing lead exposure as a starting point. Because of the temporal relationship of lead exposure to the development of hyperactivity disorder in a cohort study, one can be more confident that lead exposure is an "antecedent" or "cause." A case-control design, by contrast, would begin by identifying subjects with and without hyperactivity disorder and determining whether they had been exposed to lead. We are left with the question, "does lead exposure cause hyperactivity disorder or are children with hyperactivity disorder or a predisposition to hyperactivity disorder more likely to engage in behaviors which expose them to lead?"

In addition to its ability to confirm a sequence of events, cohort studies are less prone to several forms of bias than case-control studies. Bias in case-control studies comes primarily from two different sources:

(1) selection of cases and controls (*sampling bias*); and (2) the fact that predictor variables are being measured retrospectively.

In a cohort study, the presence or absence of disease is confirmed systematically in every patient. In a case-control study, sampling bias occurs because the cases may not be representative of people with the disease in the general population. The cases in a case-control study represent only individuals who have been diagnosed with disease. This includes people who may be misdiagnosed. It also excludes people who may have died of the disease. Survivors of disease may be healthier or may have less aggressive forms of disease than those who have died. The form of sampling bias introduced under such circumstances is called *survivor bias*. Selection of controls is also a source of sampling bias. As stated, ideally, controls would be similar to cases in every way except that they do not have disease. From a practical standpoint, finding such controls can be difficult. Imagine a study designed to determine if working in a chemical plant increases the risk of bladder cancer. One-hundred subjects with bladder cancer are recruited from a hospital urology clinic. The challenge is finding another 100 subjects who are similar but do not have bladder cancer. If 100 adults without cancer from the community at large were selected, they may differ in other important ways from the hospital clinic patients. They may be healthier in general or perhaps less health conscious in general.

Measuring predictor variables retrospectively is prone to bias. As noted, people with certain health conditions are often very conscious of past exposures and risks. In a case control study designed to determine if exposure to asbestos is associated with lung cancer, for example, the cases are likely to know more about potentially related exposures than subjects without lung cancer. This is known as *differential recall bias* and makes the association between the exposure and disease appear stronger than it really is. Researchers have ways of dealing with these two main sources of biases. (References are available in the bibliography.)

Unlike case-control studies, cohort studies are not limited to the measurement of one outcome. One can follow a cohort of patients exposed to 2,4-D, for example, and measure not only the incidence of soft-tissue sarcoma, but a number of other conditions (e.g., other cancers, emphysema, etc.). It becomes possible, therefore, to calculate multiple RRs.

The disadvantages of cohort studies compared to case-control studies relate mostly to their impracticality. Cohort studies are generally much more expensive. As noted, they are not practical for studying rare diseases or diseases which require many years to appear. Compared to randomized, controlled trials, cohort studies are more prone to confounding. In a randomized, controlled trial, the investigator not only has control over the treatment or "exposure" but can select patients to avoid potential confounders. In a cohort study, patients are defined by the exposure. Confounding variables may unknowingly influence the outcome. In a cohort study of 2,4-D, for example, it is possible that soft-tissue sarcoma is not related to 2,4-D but rather to the plants upon which the herbicide is sprayed.

PROBLEMS

1. Your colleague Domenic suspects that caffeine consumption is related to the development of glaucoma. He designs a case-control study and recruits 40 patients with glaucoma and 40 similar patients without glaucoma. Each patient is asked whether or not they drink coffee on a regular basis. Domenic's results are summarized in Table 6.5.

   Is there a significant association (with $\alpha = 0.05$) between coffee consumption and glaucoma?

2. A prospective cohort study was designed to evaluate the risk of developing pulmonary fibrosis upon exposure to fertilizer. 800 people exposed to fertilizer were compared with 800 unexposed people, and the incidence of pulmonary fibrosis was recorded over a 10-year period. Out of them, 720 people exposed to fertilizer did not develop fibrosis. There were a total of 100 cases of pulmonary fibrosis in the study. What is the RR of developing pulmonary fibrosis upon exposure to fertilizer?

3. Veterans of the 1990–1991 Gulf War appear to have an increased incidence of migraine headaches and thought to be related by some to exposure to sulfuric acid from burning refineries. Describe how you would conduct a case-control study to investigate the relationship between exposure to sulfuric acid and migraine headaches among Gulf War veterans and the challenges you might face.

TABLE 6.5   Coffee Exposure and Glaucoma

		Outcome		
		Glaucoma +	Glaucoma −	Total
Coffee drinker?	Yes	16	5	21
	No	24	35	59
Total		40	40	80

SOLUTIONS TO PROBLEMS

1. The OR is given by $\dfrac{16 \times 35}{5 \times 24} = 4.67$.

   The lower boundary of the 95% CI for this estimate is

   $$_e\ln(4.67) - 1.96 \times \sqrt{1/16 + 1/5 + 1/24 + 1/35} = 1.51.$$

   The upper boundary of the 95% CI for this estimate is

   $$_e\ln(4.67) + 1.96 \times \sqrt{1/16 + 1/5 + 1/24 + 1/35} = 14.4.$$

   The study reveals a significant association between coffee consumption and glaucoma with an OR of 4.67, 95% CI (1.51, 14.4).

2. Consider the algebraic version of the 2 × 2 table (Table 6.6) for the results of cohort studies completed with information we already know. Furthermore, we know that a must be 80 (i.e., 800 − 720). Therefore, c must be 20 (i.e., 100 − 80). We can now obtain values for all four cells in Table 6.7.

   The RR is simply $\dfrac{80/(80 + 720)}{20/(20 + 780)} = 4$.

3. The first step is to identify Gulf War veterans who suffer regularly from migraine headaches. The next step is to identify veterans that are as similar as possible to the migraine sufferers to serve as controls. They should be similar with respect to such variables as sex, age, previous history of headaches, length of deployment in the Gulf, etc. Since many soldiers served in similar environments in the Gulf, this may not be too difficult. The greater difficulty will be in ascertaining exposure to sulfuric acid. One needs to ask questions about sulfuric acid carefully and in an identical way to both cases and controls. Cases may still be more able to recall their exposure. Alternatively, if available, medical records may serve as a useful way to confirm exposure. Unfortunately many soldiers may not have sought medical attention for sulfuric acid exposure. If anamnesis is used, it may be wise to keep the soldiers naive

TABLE 6.6   Pulmonary Fibrosis and Fertilizer Exposure

		Outcome		
		Present	Absent	Total
Exposed	Yes	a	720	800
	No	c	d	800
Total		100	b + d	1600

TABLE 6.7   Pulmonary Fibrosis and Fertilizer Exposure

		Outcome		
		Present	Absent	Total
Exposed	Yes	80	720	800
	No	20	780	800
Total		100	1500	1600

to the risk factor under study. Each soldier could be asked, for example, not only about exposure to sulfuric acid, but about other types of exposures that are unrelated to migraines. Questions that are not relevant to the subject under study are known as "dummy" questions and help mitigate the problem of differential recall bias. Even with such a strategy, recall bias may be a problem. Cases may simply report being exposed to all sorts of things at a higher rate. In some case control studies, the investigators are blinded to each subjects case/control i.e., disease status. This prevents the investigators from seeking an exposure history more aggressively among the cases. Often it is hard to blind investigators to disease status, since disease status may be divulged by a study subject, or may be so obvious (e.g., amputation) that it is impossible for investigators to be blind to it.

Survival

O B J E C T I V E S

1. In general terms, describe why studying survival is complicated.
2. Define censoring, right censoring, left censoring, and interval censoring.
3. Use simple proportions and accompanying 95% CIs to summarize survival data.
4. Given a small set of survival data, use the Kaplan-Meier method to construct a survival curve.
5. Use the logrank test to identify significant differences between survival curves.
6. List three important assumptions of the Kaplan-Meier method.
7. Distinguish between survival and hazard.
8. Define hazard ratio (HR) and calculate the HR for a small set of survival data.
9. Distinguish between univariate and multivariate survival analysis.
10. In general terms, describe the Cox proportional hazards model and define the proportionality assumption.
11. Provide an interpretation of the results of a survival analysis that uses the Cox proportional hazards model.

7.1 Introduction

One of the most challenging tasks in medicine is discussing survival with a patient with a terminal illness such as advanced lung cancer. In such circumstances, patients inevitably want to know *"How long have I got doctor?"* The answer is at best an estimate based upon existing studies of similar patients with the same condition. Though *survival* refers specifically to life and death, *survival analysis*, in the context of medical decision making, refers to the length of time to any event of interest. For example, a group of women may have undergone surgical excision of nonfatal breast lumps. One may wish to know not their survival, but the amount of time to recurrence of the lumps. Survival analysis also need not necessarily refer to adverse events. The statistical procedures that are used to study and analyze data related to survival from cancer, for example, are the same procedures that are required to study and analyze data related to time to conception after treatment of fertility. For these reasons, survival analysis is more accurately described as *time-to-event analysis*. Throughout this chapter, I use the term survival analysis, since it is more familiar to most people.

7.2 Why Survival Analysis is Complicated

In Chapter 4, you learned about the design of studies of therapies. In such studies, all the patients receive one or more interventions at roughly the same time. Patients are then followed for a specific period of time, during which they may or may not experience an outcome of interest. Consider a study to evaluate the effectiveness of aspirin in preventing strokes among patients with atrial fibrillation. All patients receive either a single dose of aspirin a day or placebo. They are followed for 5 years, and the number of patients experiencing a stroke in each group is recorded. One can say that patients did or did not experience a stroke within 5 years. In survival analysis, we are interested in the amount of time to an event. Imagine that we are studying the survival of patients with atrial fibrillation who are treated with aspirin and comparing it to survival of patients treated with placebo. We cannot study all these patients forever and therefore decided that the study will last 10 years. During this time, some patients will die (from stroke or some other cause), but many will not. Among the patients who survive, we only know that they survived at least 10 years but will not know their actual survival time. We are therefore missing data about them because the event we are interested in, namely, death, has not occurred during the study. *Censoring* is the phenomenon of unknown survival times for a subset of patients under study. Censoring occurs in three ways. Usually, a patient has not experienced the event of interest (e.g., death) by the close of the study. A patient may also be lost to follow-up during the study, and his survival time will therefore be unknown. Finally, a patient may experience an event different from the one under study that makes follow-up impossible. Imagine, for example, a patient who is being followed up for lung cancer who experiences a disabling stroke and can no longer participate in a lung-cancer study.

In most cases, censoring refers to an event of interest that takes place beyond the end of the follow-up period. It is also possible in some cases that an event takes place before a follow-up period begins. Imagine a study to evaluate the time to recurrence of prostate cancer after surgical treatment. All men who had the surgery are examined 6 months after surgery. If some of them already had a recurrence at that point, it would be impossible to say exactly when the recurrence began—only that it was less than 6 months after therapy. When an event takes place beyond the end of the follow-up period, it is sometimes referred to as being *right censored*. When it takes place before the beginning of the follow-up period, it is *left censored*. *Interval censoring* refers to study subjects who come in and out of observation so that follow-up data is missing at some point in the follow-up period. Generally speaking, censoring refers to right-censored data and is the situation that will be discussed in this chapter.

There are many statistical methods used to describe survival. This chapter focuses on the most common. Some complex calculations have been deliberately omitted. As a physician or physician-in-training, it is important for you to understand the general principles of the most common methods used and how to interpret the results of such methods. More details about survival analysis can be found in sources listed in the Annotated Bibliography.

7.3 Describing Survival

CASE 7.1

Yvonne is studying the survival of patients recently diagnosed with mesothelioma, a rare and highly malignant form of lung cancer, who are treated with chemotherapy. She begins her study at the beginning of 2004 and ends it at the end of 2006. The plot next describes the survival of each of her 10 patients.

```
1 ----------------------D
                2 ----------------------------□
       3 -----------------------------D
    4 -----------D
    5 ----------------------------□
    6 ------------------------------D
    7 -------D
    8 ------------------------------------D
    9 -------------------------------D
    10 ----------D
```

JFMAMJJASOND JFMAMJJASOND JFMAMJJASOND

2004   2005   2006

"D" indicates death. "□" indicates that the data is censored. For patient 2, we know only that death takes place beyond the study period. Patient 5 was lost to follow-up in early 2005, and data about his survival is therefore unavailable. Notice that not all 10 patients were enrolled at exactly the same time. Patient 2, for example, was enrolled in the study nearly a year after it began. How can you summarize this survival data?

The first task is to convert the plot on the previous page from calendar time to time from diagnosis since this provides a more accurate picture of survival.

```
 1_____D
 2_____□
 3_____D
 4_____D
 5_____□
 6_____D
 7_____D
 8_____D
 9_____D
10_____D
 1 2 3 4 5 6 7 8 9 10 11 12 13 14 15 16 17 18 19 20 21 22 23 24 25 26 27 28 29 30 31
                              Time (months)
```

Table 7.1 shows a numerical summary of the survival times of the 10 patients:

How can we summarize this data? One simple way is to consider the proportion of patients dying within a specific time interval. Consider the

TABLE 7.1   Patients and Survival Time

Patient	Survival Time (Months)
1	18
2	Censored after 24 months
3	21
4	11
5	Censored after 15 months
6	20
7	8
8	25
9	21
10	10

proportion dying within the first year. Among 10 patients for whom we have data for at least 1 year, three died. The 1-year mortality rate or probability of dying is 3/10 (0.33 or 33%). Since survival studies make use of samples of patients just like other types of studies, this proportion of patients dying is an estimate of the proportion dying in the underlying population. The precision of this estimate can be quantified with a 95% CI given by the following formula.

$$p \pm 1.96 = \sqrt{p(1-p)/n}.$$

The formula assumes that mortality is normally distributed which may or not be true. Other formulae are used when only a very small proportion of patients or no patients experience an event in the time frame under study.

In Case 7.1, our estimate of the underlying 1-year mortality rate in the population becomes

$$0.33 \pm 1.96\sqrt{0.33(1-0.33)/10}$$

or

$$0.33, 95\% \text{ CI}(0.04, 0.62).$$

This simple analysis is somewhat useful. Survival is usually assessed with more sophisticated techniques that will be discussed in the next sections.

7.4 Kaplan-Meier Survival Estimate

The Kaplan-Meier method, also known as the product-limit method, provides us with an answer to the question, "What is the probability of survival to a certain point?" It relies on a fundamental principle of probability, namely that the probability of two independent events occurring is the product of their individual probabilities. The Kaplan-Meier method relies upon conditional probabilities. In Case 7.1, for example, the probability of surviving for 18 months is the product of surviving the first 17 months multiplied by the probability of surviving the 18th month, *given that the first 17 months were survived*. Formally, we can describe the probability of being alive at a certain time t_j by the *survivor function, $S(t_j)$* as the following:

$$S(t_j) = S(t_{j-1})(1 - d_j/n_j)$$

$S(t_{j-1})$ is the probability of being alive at time t_{j-1}, where time is measured in any unit (years, months, days, etc.), and n_j is the number of patients alive just before time t_j. d_j is the number of deaths that take place at time t_j. The value of $S(t_j)$ is constant between events, meaning for example, if nobody dies in a certain time interval, the probability of death is unchanged. At time zero, $S_{(0)}$ is equal to 1 since all patients are alive. Let us now apply this formula to the data from Case 7.1.

Yvonne's first patient died at 8 months. The probability of surviving 8 months is given by

$$S(8 \text{ months}) = 1 \times (1 - 1/10) = 0.90.$$

The next patient died at 10 months. The probability of surviving 10 months is therefore given by

$$S(10 \text{ months}) = 0.90 \times (1 - 1/9) = 0.80.$$

The next patient died at 11 months. The probability of surviving 11 months is therefore given by

$$S(11 \text{ months}) = 0.80 \times (1 - 1/8) = 0.70.$$

Patient 5 is censored after 15 months. Nothing is known after that point, therefore, about his survival. After 15 months, he is simply excluded from the analysis, as reflected by our n_j. The next death took place at 18 months. The probability of surviving 18 months is therefore given by

$$S(18 \text{ months}) = 0.70 \times (1 - 1/6) = 0.58.$$

These calculations can obviously get tedious. Most of the time they are completed using statistical software. Data is plotted to yield a *Kaplan-Meier survival curve*. A sample Kaplan-Meier curve (based on many more observations than Case 7.1) is shown in Fig. 7.1.[1]

Rituxan is a cancer drug used to treat a cancer known as non-Hodgkin's lymphoma. Figure 7.1 describes the probability of the cancer not progressing after treatment with the drug. At the time of first measurement, for example, nearly all patients are progression free. There are several other features of Fig. 7.1 that are characteristic of most survival curves. First, notice that the curve is not smooth. Survival probability decreases in a "choppy," stepwise fashion. This is because the survival function changes only when an event takes place. The probability of survival is assumed to be constant between events. Next, notice the "Cs" along the curve. This indicates points at which data is censored, i.e., patients are lost to follow-up or their survival is unknown for some other reason. Finally, notice the horizontal line originating at the point at which 50% of patients are progression free. The point at which this line intersects the survival curve indicates the *median survival*—the point at which half of patients have a probability of

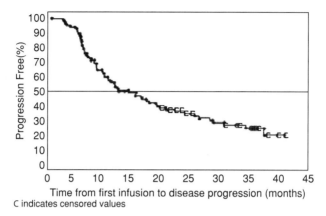

FIGURE 7.1 Sample Kaplan-Meier Curve

surviving a longer time and half a shorter time. In survival analysis, median survival is more useful than mean survival since the survival function is not usually normally distributed. In Fig. 7.1, the median survival is roughly 14 months.

As you can imagine, since the survival function in most studies is based upon samples used to estimate survival in a larger population, there is uncertainty in the estimates of survival probability at different times. It is possible to calculate a 95% CI for each estimate of survival probability and for the entire survival curve. Like survival curves, their 95% CIs are usually calculated with computers. Details about the specific calculations involved can be found in a source listed in the Annotated Bibliography. Figure 7.2 shows an example of a survival curve with 95% CI.

The dashed lines represent the 95% CI each time a new estimate of survival probability is calculated. Notice that the 95% CI becomes wider as survival probability decreases. This should be expected because the number of subjects in the sample decreases, lowering the precision of estimates of survival probability.

7.5 Comparing Survival Curves

Though single survival curves are useful, survival is usually studied as a comparison among two or more treatments or conditions. Consider Fig. 7.3 next.

It is fairly obvious that the group treated has worse survival than the control group. At every time point, survival in the control group is superior. Precise statistical methods help us answer the question, "How significant is a difference in survival curves?"

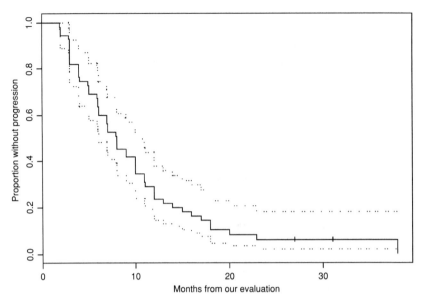

FIGURE 7.2 Kaplan-Meier Survival Curve with 95% CI

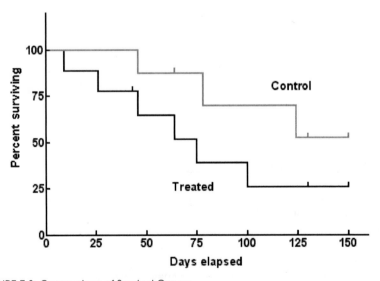

FIGURE 7.3 Comparison of Survival Curves

Astrocytoma and glioblastoma are two types of serious brain tumors. Investigators have studied the survival of women after recurrence of each of these two tumors.[2] The survival curves shown in Fig. 7.4 were obtained.

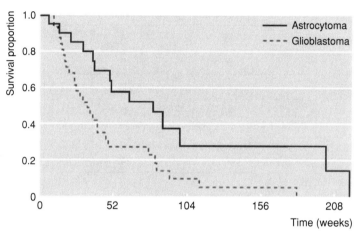

FIGURE 7.4 Survival by Tumor Type

(Reproduced with permission from Bland JM, Altman DG. The logrank test. BMJ 2004;328:1073.)

Table 7.2 shows the raw data for the weeks to death or censoring in all 51 patients studied, classified by tumor type.

TABLE 7.2   Weeks to Death or Censoring in 51 Adults with Recurrent Gliomas

A	G
6	10
13	10
21	12
30	13
31*	14
37	15
38	16
47*	17

continued

TABLE 7.2   *Continued*

A	G
49	18
50	20
63	24
79	24
80*	25
82*	28
82*	30
86	33
98	34*
149*	35
202	37
219	40
	40
	40*
	46
	48
	70*
	76
	81
	82
	91
	112
	181

A, astrocytoma; G, glioblastoma.
Reproduced with permission from Bland JM, Altman DG. The logrank test. BMJ 2004;328:1073.
*indicates that data has been censored at this point.

Is there a statistically significant difference between the two survival curves?

The simplest and most commonly used method to answer this question is the *logrank test*. It relies upon the null hypothesis that there is no difference in the probability of death at any given point between the two groups. The logrank test is a form of the χ^2 test which compares observed to expected values of the event being studied in each group. It takes the following form:

$$\chi^2 = \sum_{i=1}^{g} (O_i - E_i)^2 / E_i.$$

Here "i" represents each successive group in the study. The squared differences between the observed and expected number of events is divided by the expected number of events for each group. These values are summed across all "g" groups to yield the χ^2 statistic.

When this study started, there were a total of 51 patients: 20 patients in group "A" and 31 patients in group "G." The first patient died during week 6. The overall risk of death among all patients is therefore 1/51 at this point. If there was no difference between the risk of death between groups, the number of deaths in each group would be the following:

Group A : $1/51 \times 20 = 0.39$.

Group G : $1/51 \times 31 = 0.61$.

In week 10, two patients died, both in group G. The risk of death at this point is 2/50. The expected numbers of death in each group are respectively,

Group A : $2/50 \times 19 = 0.76$.

Group G : $2/50 \times 31 = 1.24$.

Notice that at this point there are only 19 patients in Group A. This procedure is continued until the total expected number of deaths in each group is calculated. This works out to 22.48 in group 1 and 19.52 in group 2. In Group A, 14 subjects actually died and 28 died in Group G.

χ^2 is $(14 - 22.48)^2 / 22.48 + (28 - 19.52)^2 / 19.52 = 6.88$.

There are two groups and, therefore, one degree of freedom. A χ^2 of 6.88 is associated with a p value between 0.01 and 0.005. We can conclude that if there was no significant difference between the two survival curves, the observed results would have been obtained less than 1% of the time. This is a statistically significant result.

7.6 Assumptions of the Kaplan-Meier Method

Analysis and comparison of survival curves relies upon three extremely important assumptions which must be at least approximately true in order for the analysis to be valid. First, it is assumed that patients who are censored have the same survival prospects as those who remain in a study. Imagine that the survival of patients receiving chemotherapy for lung cancer is being evaluated and a large number of patients drop out. It is possible that those who drop out have worse disease than those who remain, and therefore have a worse prognosis. Under such circumstances, the survival curve would be misleading, since it would describe better survival from disease than actually is the case. Normally, only a small number of patients are censored and censoring is not related to prognosis. This is known as *uninformative censoring*. Censoring that is related to prognosis is known as *informative censoring* and the statistical methods we have discussed are not applicable.

The next important assumption is that survival probabilities are the same for subjects recruited early in a study and late in a study. Some survival studies recruit patients over several years. Imagine that you wish to study survival among patients infected with the HIV and recruit patients between 1985 (when large numbers of patients with HIV first began to appear) and 1995. Over this 10-year period, much was learned about HIV. For example, patients with HIV disease began to be treated with antibiotics and immunizations to prevent infections which could be deadly in their immunocompromised state. Patients recruited for a survival study early on might have a worse prognosis than those recruited later, simply because patients recruited later may have been better informed, less susceptible to infection, or healthier in general for other reasons. Studying survival using a single Kaplan-Meier curve would not be valid under such circumstances since essentially, you are studying two different diseases: HIV disease in the 1980s and HIV disease in the 1990s. Two diseases should not be described with a single curve.

The final fundamental assumption is that each event that we record happens at the time specified. This is fairly straightforward for some types of unambiguous events like death, but is not always clear for other types of events such as recurrence of disease. Imagine that we wish to evaluate recurrence of prostate cancer after surgery, and assess patients every 6 months. When we find a recurrence, we assume that it occurred at that specific time, even though it may have occurred at any time in the previous 6 months. Survival probabilities would be biased upwards under such circumstances. This is usually not a huge problem. If follow-up takes place at standard, regular intervals, there are statistical methods available to account for the fact that events may take place at any point in an interval.

7.7 Survival and Hazard

Survival data can be interpreted in many ways. The survival function, as noted, describes the probability that an individual survives to a certain time. *Hazard*, by contrast, is the probability that an individual experiences an event at a specific time. Survival describes the cumulative probability of an event *not-occurring*, while hazard describes the instantaneous risk of an event *occurring*. One could say, for example, that the probability of surviving 2 years with a disease is 34% and the hazard at 2 years of dying at that point is 14%.

When two groups are being compared, we can define the *hazard ratio* (HR) as the following:

$$HR = \frac{O_1/E_1}{O_2/E_2}.$$

Here "O" represents the observed number of observations in groups 1 and 2, while "E" represents the expected number of observations in groups 1 and 2. An HR of 1 indicates no difference in overall survival between the two groups through the course of the study. A ratio below 1 indicates improved survival in group 1. A ratio above 1 indicates worse survival in group 1. An HR is therefore a type of RR. It is possible to calculate a CI for the HR to better quantify its precision and magnitude.

Construction and comparison of Kaplan-Meier curves has important limitations. First, the Kaplan-Meier method and logrank test allow us to predict and compare survival with respect to one factor only. We can construct curves for survival after two different treatments for lung cancer, for example, and compare the curves with respect to the type of treatment received only. These methods are known as *univariate analyses* since only one factor or variable is being studied at a time. More commonly, we are interested in how several different factors simultaneously influence survival. For example, in patients with lung cancer, we may be interested not only in how the treatment under study influences survival but also how other factors such as patients' age, sex, race, stage of tumor at the time of diagnosis, the presence of other diseases such as emphysema, etc. influence survival. In such cases we need *multivariate analyses* using a *multivariate model*. The most widely used such model is known as the *Cox proportional hazards model*. The general form of this model is the following:

$$h(t) = h_0(t) \times e^{(\beta_1 x_1 + \cdots + \beta_k x_k)}.$$

Here, $x_1, \ldots, x_k$ are a collection of independent variables that determine hazard such as age, sex, disease stage, etc. Variables can be continuous, categorical, or ordinal. $h_0(t)$ is the baseline hazard at time t. It is the hazard for a person who has a value of zero for all the independent variables. The quantities exp(β_k) are HRs. The Cox model is a type of regression. It relies upon one absolutely crucial assumption: *For two different patients in a study, the ratio of their hazard remains constant throughout time.* For example, let us assume we have a model that includes just three independent variables: age, sex, and race, and we wish to evaluate hazard from lung cancer, where the outcome in question is death. Through our model, we determine that a 50-year-old white male has a hazard or risk of death of 15% per year after 1 year and a 60-year-old black female has a hazard or risk of death of 10% per year at the same point. The ratio of these hazards (3:2) would remain the same after 2 years, even though the hazard associated with each patient may change. This is known as the *proportionality assumption*.

For the Cox model to be valid, the proportionality assumption must be true for each independent variable. There are many ways to test the assumption. One simple way is to look at Kaplan-Meier curves. Figure 7.5 describes the survival of kidney transplants (i.e., survival of kidneys, not of the patients) with two different immunosuppressive drugs used after transplantation.[3] In this case, the type of drug administered is an independent variable.

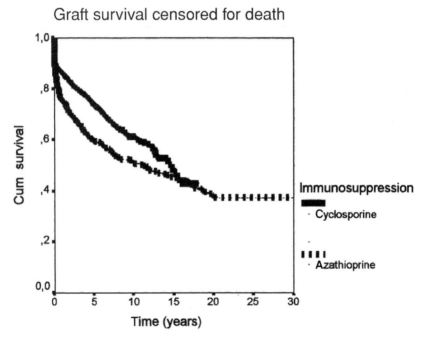

FIGURE 7.5 Graft Survival after Cyclosporine or Azathioprine

(Reproduced with permission from Roodnat JI, Mulder PGH, Tielens ETH, van Riemsdijk IC, van Gelder T, Weimar W. The Cox proportional hazards analysis in words: Examples in the renal transplantation field. Transplantation 2004;77:483–488.)

Let us say that we wish to construct a Cox model. We have two patients who are identical in every way, except with respect to the type of immunosuppressive drug each receives. At first, the patient who receives cyclosporine has a higher probability of survival and therefore a lower risk or hazard. After about 20 years, however, the two survival curves cross, as survival among patients with azathioprine and among patients with cyclosporine becomes roughly the same. When this crossing of survival curves takes place, the proportionality assumption does not hold for the independent variable in question, since the ratio of hazard throughout time was clearly not constant.

Also in order to be valid, a Cox model should not include an indefinite number of variables. In general, the number of variables in a Cox model should be no more than 10% of the total number of events that takes place or the square root of the number of events, whichever is lower. A Cox model of a survival study that includes 100 deaths, for example, should include no more than 10 variables (age, sex, disease status, etc.).

The Cox model itself may seem somewhat abstract at this point. Furthermore, the details about how the Cox model is constructed, including calculations of the individual HRs (βs), also known as *coefficients* are complex and cumbersome. Cox models are normally constructed using sophisticated statistical software programs. For your purposes, it is important for you to understand what the Cox proportional hazards model is and how it is used. It is also important to be able to interpret the results of the application of such a model when you encounter it in the medical literature.

CASE 7.3

Peritoneal kidney dialysis is often sometimes associated with a serious infection called peritonitis. Recently, Chinese investigators developed a Cox proportional hazards model to explain the factors associated with development of peritonitis.[4] Their results are shown in Table 7.3.

TABLE 7.3   Independent Predictors of Dialysis-Associated Peritonitis, According to a Multivariate Cox Regression Analysis

	HR (95% CI) of Developing Peritonitis	p Value
Diabetes mellitus	2.08 (0.88–4.95)	0.096
Baseline serum albumin concentration (every 10g/L decrease)	1.80 (0.68–4.80)	0.242
Age < 40 years	2.87 (0.80–10.30)	0.348

continued

TABLE 7.3   *Continued*

	HR (95% CI) of Developing Peritonitis	p Value
Receiving social security assistance	2.69 (1.10–6.54)	0.029
Illiterate subjects	2.73 (1.04–7.20)	0.041

How would you interpret these results?

First, notice that the HRs are accompanied by 95% CIs. An HR of 1.0 indicates that presence of the factor does not increase or decrease the hazard. A 95% CI that includes 1.0, therefore, indicates that the associated factor is not statistically significant. The results also include p values. At a level of significance of 0.05, the only significant HRs are for the factors, "receiving social security assistance" and "illiterate subjects." The HRs can be interpreted in the following way: the hazard for developing peritonitis is 2.69 times higher among patients receiving social security assistance than patients not receiving social security assistance, and 2.73 times higher among illiterate subjects than non-illiterate subjects.

PROBLEMS

1. Amyotrophic lateral sclerosis (ALS) is a fatal, progressive neurological disease. Table 7.4 shows the survival times from the time of diagnosis of 10 patients with ALS collected during a 10-year study. Construct a Kaplan-Meier curve based on this data and provide an approximate value for the median survival.

2. Complex pulmonary atresia is a serious congenital condition in which the blood supply to the lungs is abnormal. Survival among patients with this condition is thought to depend upon whether they have normal pulmonary artery anatomy or not, at the time of presentation. Table 7.5 shows the data on the survival in days of 30 patients with complex pulmonary atresia based on whether they have normal pulmonary artery anatomy (pa-anat = 1) or abnormal anatomy (pa-anat = 0).[5] Calculate the overall HR for abnormal versus normal pulmonary artery anatomy.

3. Table 7.6 shows the results of a Cox proportional hazards analysis of failure of an organ after transplantation (i.e., the endpoint is failure of the organ transplanted, not death).[5] What conclusions can you draw from these results?

TABLE 7.4   Survival Among Patients with ALS

Patient No.	Survival Time (Years)
1	8.3
2	Censored after 3.5 years
3	3.0
4	5.0
5	Censored after 10 years
6	4.3
7	5.5
8	9.0
9	4.0
10	4.5

SOLUTIONS TO PROBLEMS

1. Recall that we describe the probability of surviving to a certain time with the formula

$$S(t_j) = S(t_{j-1})(1 - d_j/n_j).$$

Table 7.7 shows the data arranged according to survival time.
The first patient died at 3 years. The probability of surviving 3 years is given by

$$1 \times (1 - 1/10) = 0.90.$$

Using the same procedure, we can construct the values as shown in Table 7.8 for the survival function:
Note that two values are censored. We know that patient 5 survived the full 10 years of the study but we do not know his total survival time. The corresponding Kaplan-Meier curve is shown in Fig. 7.6. The median survival is approximately 5 years.

2. It is necessary to calculate the total number of observed and expected number of deaths in each group to calculate the HR. Recall that

$$HR = \frac{O_1/E_1}{O_2/E_2}.$$

TABLE 7.5   Normal or Abnormal Pulmonary Artery Anatomy and Survival Time

Patient ID No.	Event Time	Pa-anat=0		Pa-anat=1	
		At Risk	Observed	At Risk	Observed
5	4	20	1	10	0
15	14	19	1	10	0
21	88	19	0	9	1
3	117	16	1	9	0
2	121	16	0	8	1
30	142	16	0	7	1
29	193	16	0	6	1
14	247	16	0	5	1
17	275	14	1	5	0
12	393	13	1	5	0
28	1100	13	0	4	1
16	1791	9	1	4	0
24	2982	9	0	3	1
11	3098	5	1	3	0

At 4 days, one patient died in the abnormal pulmonary artery anatomy group (pa-anat = 0). There are a total of 30 patients in both groups. If there was no difference in the death rate between groups, we would expect 1/30 patients in each group to die.

$$[\text{Pa-anat} = 0] \ (1/30 \times 20) = 0.667,$$
$$[\text{Pa-anat} = 1] \ (1/30 \times 10) = 0.333.$$

Similarly, we can calculate the expected number of deaths in each group with each event (in this case, death). Table 7.9 includes both the observed and expected values.[5]
For Pa-anat = 0, the total number of observed deaths is 7. The total expected number is 10.438. For Pa-anat = 1, the observed number is 8,

TABLE 7.6   Cox Proportional Hazards Analysis of Organ Failure after Transplantation

	Exp(B)	95% CI for Exp(B)	p	p
Graft failure censored for death				
Recipient age (per year)	0.98	0.96–0.99	0.0002	
Donor gender (female)	1.33	1.10–1.60	0.0030	
Type of immunosuppression (CsA)	0.78	0.53–1.15	NS	0.0031
Type of immunosuppression × time (time ≥ 4 year)	2.13	1.37–3.32	0.0009	

CsA, cyclosporine A; NS, not significant; Exp(B), exponent of the B-coefficient.
Reproduced with permission from Roodnat JI, Mulder PGH, Tielens ETH, van Riemsdijk IC, van Gelder T, Weimar W. The Cox proportional hazards analysis in words: Examples in the renal transplantation field. Transplantation 2004;77:483–488.

TABLE 7.7   Data Arranged According to Survival Time

Patient No.	Survival Time (Years)
3	3.0
2	Censored after 3.5 years
9	4.0
6	4.3
10	4.5
4	5.0
7	5.5
1	8.3
8	9.0
5	Censored after 10 years

TABLE 7.8   Survival Time and Values of Survival Function

Survival Time (Years)	Survival Function S(*t*)
3.0	$1 \times (1 - 1/10) = 0.90$
4.0	$0.90 \times (1 - 1/8) = 0.79$
4.3	$0.79 \times (1 - 1/7) = 0.68$
4.5	$0.68 \times (1 - 1/6) = 0.57$
5.0	$0.57 \times (1 - 1/5) = 0.46$
5.5	$0.46 \times (1 - 1/4) = 0.35$
8.3	$0.35 \times (1 - 1/3) = 0.23$
9.0	$0.23 \times (1 - 1/2) = 0.12$

while the expected number is 4.561. The HR is therefore,

$$HR = \frac{8/4.561}{7/10.438} = 2.615.$$

3. The Exp(B) values represent HRs. The 95% CIs and p values indicate that only 3 of 4 of these ratios are statistically significant. For recipient

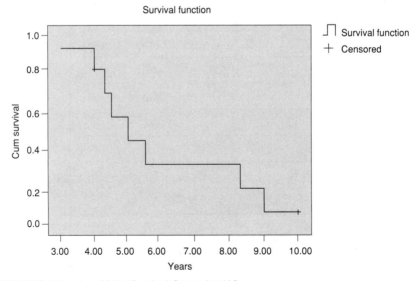

FIGURE 7.6 Kaplan–Meier Survival Curve for ALS

TABLE 7.9

Patient	Event Time	Pa-anat=0			Pa-anat=1		
		At Risk	Observed	Expected	At Risk	Observed	Expected
5	4	20	1	0.667	10	0	0.333
15	14	19	1	0.655	10	0	0.345
21	77	19	0	0.655	9	1	0.345
19	88	19	0	0.678	9	1	0.321
3	117	16	1	0.640	9	0	0.360
2	121	16	0	0.667	8	1	0.333
30	142	16	0	0.696	7	1	0.304
29	193	16	0	0.727	6	1	0.273
14	247	16	0	0.762	5	1	0.238
17	275	14	1	0.737	5	0	0.263
12	393	13	1	0.722	5	0	0.278
28	1100	13	0	0.765	4	1	0.235
16	1791	9	1	0.692	4	0	0.308
24	2982	9	0	0.750	3	1	0.250
11	3098	5	1	0.625	3	0	0.375

age we can conclude that the graft failure rate decreases with advancing age. Specifically, for each extra year of age, the hazard of graft failure decreases by $1 - 0.98 = 0.02$, or 2%. The hazard associated with being female versus being male is 1.33 (or 33% higher). The type of immunosuppression (cyclosporine versus azathioprine) does not yield a statistically significant HR, but C_sA administration for 4 years or more does significantly increase the hazard more than twofold over baseline.

References

1. McLaughlin P. Rituximab Investigator's Meeting, Seattle, Wash, August 1999. URL: www.rituxan.com/rituxan/professional/use/experience/relapsed/progression.jsp. Accessed December 29, 2005.

2. Bland JM, Altman DG. The logrank test. *BMJ* 2004;328:1073.
3. Roodnat JI, Mulder PGH, Tielens ETH, van Riemsijk IC, van Gelder T, Weimar W. The Cox proportional hazards analysis in words: Example in the renal transplantation field. *Transplantation* 2004;77:483–488.
4. Chow KM, Szeto CC, Leung CB, Law MC, Li PK. Impact of social factors on patients on peritoneal dialysis. *Nephrol Dial Transplant* 2005;20(11): 2504–2510.
5. Bull K, Spiegelhalter DJ. Tutorial in biostatistics. Survival analysis in observational studies. *Stat Med* 1997;16:1041–1074.

Systematic Reviews

O B J E C T I V E S

1. Define the terms narrative review, systematic review, qualitative systematic review, and quantitative systematic review (meta-analysis).
2. List the steps involved in the development of a systematic review.
3. As they apply to systematic reviews, define the terms heterogeneity, clinical heterogeneity, methodological heterogeneity, and statistical heterogeneity.
4. In general terms, describe Cochran's Q statistic to measure statistical heterogeneity.
5. In general terms, describe inconsistency and its advantages over Cochran's Q.
6. Distinguish between the fixed effects and random effects model for pooling results across studies for a quantitative systematic review.
7. Calculate the variance of a 2×2 table.
8. Combine the results of several studies in the form of 2×2 tables using either a fixed or random effects method to yield a summary OR accompanied by a 95% CI.
9. Explain sensitivity analysis as it applies to systematic reviews.
10. Define publication bias and citation bias.
11. Describe how funnel plots can be used to detect publication bias or bias in locating studies in the development of systematic reviews.

8.1 Introduction

In Chapter 4, the origins of the modern clinical trial were discussed. James Lind randomly selected pairs of sailors to receive different treatments for scurvy. What is especially important for this chapter is the title of his paper based on this study:

A Treatise of the Scurvy in Three Parts. Containing an Inquiry into the Nature, Causes and Cure of that Disease, Together with a Critical and Chronological View of what has been published on the subject.[1]

185

Lind's paper included a critical review of what had been previously published. He went about this task methodically or *systematically*. A systematic review is a form of original research whose purpose is to answer a precisely defined clinical question through careful identification, critical appraisal, and analysis of previously published literature that addresses the question. The methods used are explicit and reproducible, meaning that it is possible for someone besides the author or authors of a systematic review to use the same methodology and obtain exactly the same results. Systematic reviews use data about subjects in individual studies, but the subjects for a systematic review are essentially the studies themselves. There are two basic types. A *qualitative systematic review* is a paper in which individual studies are identified, appraised, summarized, and analyzed individually. Conclusions are based upon an overall qualitative (as opposed to statistical or quantitative) analysis of the individual studies. A *quantitative systematic review* includes all the elements of a qualitative systematic review but some or all data from individual studies is combined through explicit statistical methods to generate a summary or "pooled" result. Quantitative systematic reviews are more commonly referred to as *meta-analyses*.

It is important to distinguish systematic reviews from *narrative reviews*. A narrative review is simply a summary of what is important about a particular topic or the latest developments in a particular area. Narrative reviews do not usually address a specific clinical question. Typically an editor will ask an expert to prepare a narrative review. In theory, the experts should be unbiased in how they prepare the review. In practice, most experts who write narrative reviews already have an idea of what they wish to write, what evidence is relevant, and what recommendations should be incorporated into clinical practice. Narrative reviews, therefore, are prone to bias and more likely to reflect the opinions of the author than conclusions drawn from an exhaustive review of the literature.

Systematic reviews evolved out of necessity and have become an important part of the medical literature for several reasons. First, hundreds of new studies are published each year. A single clinical question may be addressed by several of them. Moreover, different studies frequently report conflicting results. Systematic reviews synthesize evidence from individual studies into a more digestible form. Rather than reading several papers that address a single question and attempting to draw conclusions from potentially conflicting results, a clinician can refer to a single systematic review in which the work of synthesis and interpretation has already been done.

The presence of studies that address the same question but yield conflicting results points to another important need for systematic reviews. Although hundreds of clinical trials of therapies, for example, are published annually, the number of very large clinical trials that address important questions is relatively small. Such clinical trials cost millions of dollars.

Most studies of therapies have relatively small sample sizes. As you have learned, the smaller the sample size, the lower is the power of a study. Individual studies with low power are generally not useful in medical decision making. Conflicting results among studies addressing the same question are often the result of studies with different levels of power; some are able to detect a difference between therapies, while others are not. The process of meta-analysis involves pooling results across studies. This has the potential not only to increase power, but also to increase the precision of a result. Meta-analyses (quantitative systematic reviews), therefore, provide a more accurate picture than individual small studies.

Preparation of a systematic review involves a rigorous attempt to identify all potential evidence and critical appraisal of papers that meet strict criteria. This process often reveals serious shortcomings in the medical literature. Systematic reviews set out to find answers to important clinical questions. Conclusions of systematic reviews often take the form, "The number of high quality studies that address this question is small. It is impossible for us to recommend for or against treatment A versus treatment B."

While a conclusion of this type is not useful in making clinical decisions, it brings to light the need for good quality studies that address the question. Systematic reviews, therefore, can pinpoint important gaps in research that can be addressed through new studies.

8.2 Finding and Processing Evidence

Finding evidence for a systematic review is similar to finding evidence that addresses any specific clinical question. In general, however, systematic reviewers are more thorough in their search. Clinical questions are answered by interpreting the *best* available evidence. Such evidence usually comes from original studies in leading journals. The best evidence is unlikely to be unpublished or unavailable in a common electronic database such as Medline. Systematic reviews, by contrast, attempt to answer questions based on *all* the available evidence. Indeed, one of the criteria that determines the quality of a systematic review is the thoroughness of the search for evidence. To be thorough, systematic reviewers not only search all relevant electronic databases, but also the reference lists at the end of all articles they retrieve. They also contact experts in the field to find out any evidence that their search may have missed (including unpublished studies).

Systematic reviewers establish inclusion and exclusion criteria for articles, much the same way as investigators initiating a clinical trial establish inclusion or exclusion criteria for patients. They may choose to include studies that use only a specific design or include only certain types of patients or a minimum sample size. Typically, a large number of articles are retrieved but only a handful are included for review because the majority do not meet the inclusion criteria.

Once a set of articles for review has been assembled, the next step is to determine the quality of the articles. This is a critical step. A systematic review is only as good and as useful as its constituent articles. If the evidence available to answer a clinical question is poor, a systematic review of the evidence will also be poor. A number of methods of grading quality are available and very easy to use. Worksheets from the *User's Guide to the Medical Literature* are widely used. A different worksheet is used depending upon where an article falls into the EBM paradigm. Articles that do not meet a certain number of quality criteria are excluded. Alternatively, a quality score can be assigned to each article. A minimum score can be a requirement for being included for review.

The procedures for finding and processing evidence are usually described succinctly in a systematic review, but in enough detail to be reproducible. The following is an example accompanied by a description of the articles found.[2]

> Four of the authors (GR, LF, TO, and CE) performed independent searches of the Medline database (1966–2001), using a number of medical subject headings (*exp tremor, exp PD, essential tremor*) combined with the search terms and strategy used for the *Rational Clinical Examination* series of articles.
>
> All relevant articles were retrieved. The resulting set of articles was divided into three parts, each of which was reviewed by a pair of authors. The reference lists of all articles were also carefully searched for additional articles. Articles were included for study if they met the following criteria: dealt primarily with the diagnosis of PD; included patients presenting with one or more typical Parkinsonian symptoms or signs (e.g., tremor, rigidity); final diagnosis confirmed by a suitable criteria standard, such as serial or detailed neurological evaluation or pathological confirmation at autopsy; and contained original data from which 2×2 tables could be extracted to calculate the sensitivity, specificity, and positive and negative LRs for different signs and symptoms. As the number of suitable articles was small, additional inclusion criteria such as a minimum sample size or publication after a certain year were not used. However, the quality of articles included was assessed according to criteria previously developed for this series.

8.3 Abstracting of Data

Data from individual studies is assembled in two forms. Summaries of qualitative information include such things as each study's patient demographics, type of intervention, year published, etc. Quality scores, if available, can also be included with this information. Table 8.1 is an example of

TABLE 8.1   Studies Included in Systematic Review

Grade C Studies Induced for Review

Source	No. of Subjects	Age, Mean (Range), y	Patient Population	Reference Standard for Diagnosis of PD	Reason Study Not Grade A
Hughes et al. 1992	100	64.5 (31–85)	Diagnosed clinically as having PD	Autopsy findings of depletion of nigral pigmented neurons and proliferation of Lewy bodies	Significant selection bias because patients studied were clinically diagnosed as having PD
Wenning et al. 2000	138	60.6 (NA)	Diagnosed clinically as having PD or MSA	Autopsy findings consistent with PD or MSA	Significant selection bias because patients studied were clinically diagnosed as having PD or MSA
Pearce et al. 1968	100	47.8 (NA)	Unselected impatients and outpatients diagnosed as having PD and controls without known neurological disease	Detailed neurological examination	Samples of patients who obviously have the condition; comparisons nonindependent; small sample size
Duarte et al. 1995	128	66.3 (30–89)*	Patients attending a movement disorders polyclinic for the first time	Detailed neurological evaluation	Convenience sample including many individuals likely to have PD; small sample size
Mutch et al. 1991	123				Nonindependent comparisons with unclear standard: samples of patients who obviously have the condition: small sample size
Cases		75 (57–89)	35 diagnosed as having PD	Unclear standard used	
Controls		73 (71–76)	88 from general practices	Neurological evaluation	
Meneghini et al. 1992	108	NA	87 inpatients with neurological disorders and 21 patients without known neurological disease	Detailed neurological evaluation	Samples of patients who obviously have the condition (including many individuals likely to have PD and controls); small sample size; prone to observer bias

PD, Parkinson disease; MSA, multisystem atrophy; NA, not available.

* For 37 patients diagnosed as having PD only.

Reproduced with permission from Rao G, Fisch L, Srinivasan S, Damico F, Okada T, Eaton C, et al. Does this patient have Parkinson disease? JAMA 2003;289(3):350.

such qualitative information summarized for the same systematic review whose search methods were described earlier.

Quantitative information is summarized separately and includes measures of the effect of a therapy, the quality of a diagnostic test, etc. If possible, the statistic used to summarize the main result of one paper should be the same for all papers. For example, in a systematic review of cohort studies examining the association between carbon tetrachloride exposure and bladder cancer, if some papers report RRs and others report ORs, one should choose one statistic or the other and summarize the results of all papers with the same statistic. This often involves "delving" in to each paper to obtain the necessary data.

CASE 8.1

Gustav is in the process of systematically reviewing the literature to answer the question, how useful is ultrasound in the diagnosis of rotator cuff tears of the shoulder? Four papers meet his inclusion criteria. The main results of the four papers are shown in Table 8.2.

TABLE 8.2   Summary of Results of Studies to be Included in Systematic Review

Paper	Main Result		
1. Wickam et al. (1998)	Gold standard (MRI)		
	U/S	+	−
	+	90	5
	−	10	95
2. Banerjee et al. (2006)	LR(+) = 14.0; LR (−) = 0.2		
3. Boynhaus and Friedman (2003)	LR(+) = 8.0; LR (−) = 0.4		
4. Cunningham (2000)	Sensitivity of ultrasound = 75%; specificity, 50%		

How would you summarize these results in a uniform fashion?

These four results should be summarized with either sensitivity/specificity or LRs. Paper 1 provides a 2×2 table from which either LRs or sensitivity/specificity can be calculated. Assuming papers 2 and 3 provide only LRs without any 2×2 tables, it is not possible to calculate sensitivity or specificity. In paper 4, however, LRs can be calculated using sensitivity and specificity. LRs, therefore, are the appropriate way to summarize this data.

1. Wickham et al. $LR(+) = 90/100|1 - 95/100 = 18$; $LR(-) = 1 - 90/100|95/100 = 0.1$.

2. Banerjee et al. $LR(+) = 14$; $LR(-) = 0.2$.

3. Boynhaus and Friedman $LR(+) = 8.0$; $LR(-) = 0.4$.

4. Cunningham $LR(+) = 0.75/1 - 0.5 = 1.5$; $LR(-) = 1 - 0.75/0.5 = 0.5$

8.4 Qualitative and Quantitative Summaries

Once data has been abstracted, the next step is to decide whether to draw conclusions based on a qualitative assessment of the data or to combine or "pool" results from one or more studies into a meta-analysis. A qualitative assessment includes descriptive statements about the papers and their results. For Case 8.1, for example, a description could read, "Among four methodologically sound studies, the positive LRs for ultrasound in the detection of rotator cuff tears range from 1.5 to 18; the negative LRs range from 0.1 to 0.5. Despite this wide variation, it is possible to conclude that ultrasound is a useful tool for the detection of rotator cuff tears."

In reality, most statistical outcomes of studies, as they are based upon samples, are accompanied by some measure of imprecision or certainty such as CIs or p values. CIs would accompany the LRs for ultrasound described before, for example. CIs are generally preferred to p values. One effective form of quantitative summary seen primarily in meta-analyses but also found in qualitative systematic reviews is known as a *forest plot*. A forest plot is a quantitative summary of the principal results of the studies included for review. An example is shown in Figure 8.1.[3]

This is a meta-analysis of the effect of the drug acetyl cysteine for prevention of kidney failure after a diagnostic procedure known as intravascular angiography. An OR of 1.23 in Figure 8.1, for example, means that the odds of developing kidney failure after administration of acetyl cysteine are 1.23 times higher than the odds of developing kidney failure without administration of acetyl cysteine, among patients who undergo intravascular angiography. The details of the specific purpose of the meta-analysis are not important for the time being. This forest plot is typical of most you will encounter in the medical literature.

The left hand column is a list of the principal authors of each of the studies included for review. The vertical line in the center of the plot represents "no difference" between the treatment being evaluated and some other treatment (in this case placebo). This meta-analysis uses ORs. An OR of 1.0 represents "no difference." No difference between two therapies could also be represented by a RR of 1.0 or an absolute difference of zero. The dark rectangular boxes represent the relative weight of each study in the meta-analysis. As will be discussed in more detail, large, precise studies receive a higher weight than small imprecise studies. A larger box usually means a larger sample size. The horizontal lines that emanate from

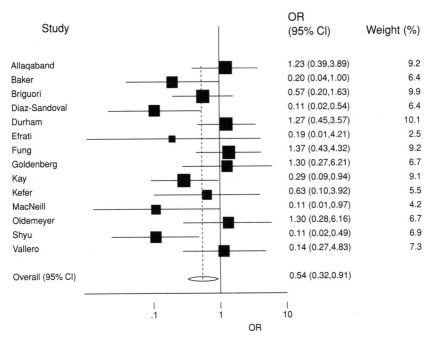

FIGURE 8.1 Sample Forest Plot

(Reproduced from Bagshaw SM, Ghali WA. Acetylcysteine for prevention of contrast-induced nephropathy after intravascular angiography: A systematic review and meta-analysis. BMC Med 2004;2:38.)

each rectangle define the 95% CI for the ORs for each study. The study by Elfrati, for example, has a very wide CI. Its OR is a very imprecise estimate. Note that the CI for all but one of the studies cross the line of no difference (OR of 1.0). The ORs and weights for each study are shown on the right of the graph.

Turn your attention to the hollow flattened diamond at the bottom of the forest plot. It represents the overall or combined or "pooled" effect. In this case, the pooled OR is 0.54. The ORs from the individual studies have been statistically combined. This, of course, is the fundamental difference between a meta-analysis and a qualitative systematic review. How a pooled result is calculated will be discussed later.

8.5 Heterogeneity

Heterogeneity can be defined as any type of variability among studies in a systematic review. There are three types of such variability. Variability in the subjects studied, interventions, or outcomes among the studies included for a review is called *clinical heterogeneity* or *clinical diversity*. In Case 8.1, for example, two of the studies may have included only patients over the age of 50 whereas the other two included patients of all ages. Alternatively, two of the studies may have included only patients with severe shoulder symptoms who are more likely to have severe and more easily detectable rotator cuff tears. Variability in the design or quality of studies is referred to as *methodological heterogeneity* or *methodological diversity*. An example of methodological diversity from a systematic review of clinical trials of a therapy might be the use of double blinding in some of the trials but not others. Finally, *statistical heterogeneity* is the observation that the observed differences in treatment effects among studies in a systematic review are greater than those one would expect on the basis of random error. When you see the term heterogeneity by itself in the medical literature, it usually refers to statistical heterogeneity.

When there is a great deal of clinical or methodological heterogeneity, results should not be statistically combined from different studies. This makes sense intuitively. In Case 8.1, for example, if studies of patients with very severe shoulder symptoms are combined with the other studies, the pooled LR would be a misleading measure of the usefulness of ultrasound in diagnosis. Ultrasound may be useful in detecting very severe rotator cuff tears but less useful in detecting the types of tears one most often encounters in clinical practice. Combining the studies together may make ultrasound seem more useful than is the case in most clinical settings. Essentially, one cannot combine apples and oranges and draw reasonable conclusions. Similarly, if studies are heterogeneous with respect to design and quality, it is inappropriate to combine them together. Such studies address the same question through different methods, and it is unsurprising that the answers also differ. Combined results in such cases are not meaningful. Consider the following analogy: Two people are asked to find out how long it takes to build a chair. The first is given only hand tools. The second is given a complete workshop of electrical tools. The first reports that it takes 40 hours to build a chair, while the second reports it to be just 4 hours. We should not average these numbers together to obtain a mean time of 22 hours. That length of time does not accurately represent anyone's time required to build a chair.

Assuming that clinical and methodological heterogeneity are not concerns, we are left with the issue of statistical heterogeneity. This remains an area of controversy. Some believe that combining results that are statistically very heterogeneous is inappropriate. More commonly, the thinking is that statistical heterogeneity is inevitable in systematic reviews and should not prevent a systematic reviewer from pooling results across studies. How can statistical heterogeneity be measured? Visual inspection of a forest plot is the simplest way. Look at Figures 8.2 and 8.3 next. In Figure 8.2, there is considerable overlap among the CIs of the different studies. By

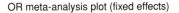

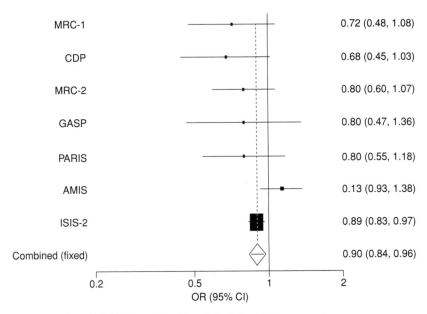

FIGURE 8.2 Forest Plot Without Significant Statistical Heterogeneity

contrast, in Figure 8.3, it is obvious that there is a little such overlap. The studies comprising the systematic review in Figure 8.3 are clearly more statistically heterogeneous.

There are more sophisticated ways of measuring statistical heterogeneity. For many years, *Cochran's Q statistic* was widely used as a measure. You need no more than a basic understanding of where Q comes from. In general terms, to calculate Cochran's Q, results across studies are statistically pooled to yield a summary estimate (i.e., diamonds in Figures 8.1–8.3). Then the squared deviations of each study's estimate of effect from the overall effect are summed while each study is weighted appropriately. This yields the Q statistic. Pooling and weighting will be discussed in the next section. The Q statistic is then compared to the χ^2 distribution with $k - 1$ degrees of freedom to obtain a p value, where k is the number of studies. If the p value is statistically significant (say at a level of 0.05), there is significant statistical heterogeneity. Several different formulae for the Q statistic are used, depending upon the method of pooling and the type of outcome measure. One formula for Q when the measures of effect are expressed as ORs is as follows.

$$Q = \Sigma w_i [(\ln OR_i) - (\ln OR_{overall})]^2,$$

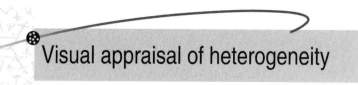

Zinc for common cold:
Summary and incidence OR for the incidence of any cold symptom at 1 week

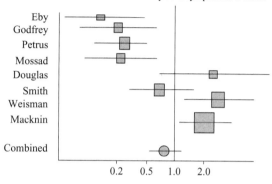

FIGURE 8.3 Forest Plot With Significant Heterogeneity

(Reproduced with permission from Jackson JL, Lesho E, Peterson C. Zinc and the common cold: A meta-analysis revisited. J Nutr 2000;130(5S Suppl):1512S–1515S.)

where w_i is the weight assigned to the ith study. ln OR_i is the natural log of the OR of the ith study.

The Q statistic has some important shortcomings. The significance of Q depends upon the number of studies included in a meta-analysis. When the number of studies is low, Q has low power to detect heterogeneity. When the number of studies is high, Q is often significant despite relatively low levels of heterogeneity. For these reasons, the Cochrane Collaboration, a network of researchers who publish high-quality systematic reviews, now uses a different statistic to measure "consistency" or "inconsistency" among the studies included in a meta-analysis, designated I^2. I^2 is calculated using the Q statistic as follows.

$$I^2 = 100\% \times (Q - \mathrm{df})/Q,$$

where df is the number of degrees of freedom (number of studies included for review − 1). Thus I^2 can be defined as the percentage of the variability in effect among studies that is due to statistical heterogeneity rather than chance. Values of I^2 greater than 50% are considered to represent high levels of statistical heterogeneity.

I^2 has significant advantages over Q. First, it yields a percentage rather than a number accompanied by a p value. It tells us, therefore, more than whether there is significant heterogeneity or not. Second, I^2 is more versatile. It provides a reliable measure of heterogeneity among systematic reviews with different numbers of studies and can be interpreted in a similar way regardless of the type of outcome data (e.g., continuous, categorical) or effect measure (e.g., OR, RR) used. Furthermore, I^2 can be accompanied by a 95% CI, which provides a range of the degree of statistical heterogeneity or "inconsistency" in a systematic review.

As noted, statistical heterogeneity is no longer considered to be a reason not to pool results together. Indeed, a high level of I^2 raises new and important questions. What appears to be significant statistical heterogeneity may actually represent clinical heterogeneity. A high I^2 also may indicate methodological heterogeneity that has been overlooked. A couple of lower quality studies included in a meta-analysis, for example, could contribute to a high I^2. Some of the studies included in a meta-analysis may have included patients that differed in significant ways from the patients in other studies. I^2 actually alerts a systematic reviewer to examine such questions.

8.6 Principles of Pooling Results

The previous sections mentioned pooled effect measures and weighting. How does one pool results from different studies to obtain an overall measure? It is tempting to simply average all the results together. For example, if a systematic review includes 10 studies and 10 ORs, one would simply add up the ORs and divide by 10. This is not appropriate because some studies are larger than others or more precise than others. They should contribute more to the overall measure than smaller, less precise studies. This is why measures of effect are weighted. There are also two different statistical techniques for combining results that rely upon different assumptions. The *fixed effects model* assumes that all the studies in a meta-analysis are estimating precisely the same effect and any variability in results is due only to random variation. According to this model, therefore, if all the studies were infinitely large, they would give identical results. This model is designed to measure this single common effect. The *random effects model* assumes that each study is estimating a different underlying effect and takes this assumption into consideration in calculating an overall effect. According to this model, the effects from different studies are randomly distributed. It provides an estimate of the center point of this distribution. For the same meta-analysis, the fixed effects model yields an overall effect measure with narrower confidence intervals than the random effects model.

The choice of model is somewhat arbitrary and remains a source of controversy. If there is no statistical heterogeneity, the fixed and random effects models yield roughly the same values for an overall effect, since the fixed effects model does not take statistical heterogeneity into account. When there is a high level of statistical heterogeneity, it is more appropriate to use the random effects model. In both models, studies are weighted by some measure of their sample size and/or variance (precision).

8.7 Fixed Effects Methods

There are three popular specific fixed effect methods for pooling results: the inverse variance method, the Mantel–Haenszel method, and Peto method. The choice of method depends upon several different factors: (1) Only the inverse variance method allows combining of continuous data; (2) The Mantel–Haenszel method is best when the number of studies is small or the size of each study is small; (3) Both the inverse variance and Mantel–Haenszel methods are used to combine ORs or other statistics derived from 2 × 2 tables; (4) Only the Peto method can be used when one of the cells of a 2 × 2 table in a study is 0. The calculations involved are similar in all three methods. It is important for you to understand the general principles in the calculations. Details of all three methods can be found elsewhere. The inverse variance method for dichotomous data is illustrated for Case 8.2.

CASE 8.2

Marlene has obtained results from three papers she wishes to combine for a meta-analysis. The question she wishes to address is whether daily aspirin therapy is protective against deep venous thrombosis among patients who have just undergone major surgery. She extracts the data necessary from the three papers to construct three 2 × 2 contingency tables (Tables 8.3–8.5).

TABLE 8.3   Webster et al. (2006)

	Deep Venous Thrombosis	No Deep Venous Thrombosis	Total
Aspirin	6	118	124
No aspirin	18	104	122
Total	24	222	246

TABLE 8.4   Mattanio et al. (2003)

	Deep Venous Thrombosis	No Deep Venous Thrombosis	Total
Aspirin	9	61	70
No aspirin	12	58	70
Total	21	119	140

TABLE 8.5   Xu and Nielson (2000)

	Deep Venous Thrombosis	No Deep Venous Thrombosis	Total
Aspirin	2	28	30
No aspirin	3	27	30
Total	5	55	60

Provide an overall measure of the effect of aspirin on the prevention of deep venous thrombosis after surgery.

To understand the inverse variance method, let us return to the general algebraic form of a 2×2 contingency table (Table 8.6).

TABLE 8.6   Algebraic 2 × 2 Contingency Table

a_i	b_i
c_i	d_i

Since we will be combining results from multiple tables, the subscript "i" represents the ith table.

The OR for this table is given by

$$OR_i = \frac{a_i d_i}{b_i c_i}.$$

The "summary" or "pooled" OR is given by the following formula.

$$\ln OR_{\text{Overall}} = \frac{\sum w_i \ln OR_i}{\sum w_i}.$$

The "w" stands for "weight." The OR from each study is weighted by the inverse of its variance. This makes sense. Studies that have a great deal of variability or variance should contribute less to the overall OR. Such studies are generally of lower sample size. More precise studies, with less variance, should contribute more:

$$w_i = 1/\mathrm{var}_i$$

Var_i is the variance of a 2×2 table which is given by the sum of the inverses of the values in each cell.

$$\mathrm{Var}_i = \frac{1}{a_i} + \frac{1}{b_i} + \frac{1}{c_i} + \frac{1}{d_i}.$$

For Webster et al., the OR is 0.29 and ln OR $= -1.22$; w is $1/0.24 = 4.16$.
For Mattanio et al., the OR is 0.71 and ln OR $= -0.34$; w is $1/0.23 = 4.38$.
For Xu and Nielson, the OR is 0.64 and ln OR $= -0.44$; w is $1/0.91 = 1.10$.

$$\ln \mathrm{OR}_{\mathrm{Overall}} = \frac{(-1.22 \times 4.16) + (-0.34 \times 4.38) + (-0.44 \times 1.10)}{4.16 + 4.38 + 1.10} = -0.731.$$

The $\mathrm{OR}_{\mathrm{Overall}} = 0.48$.

The odds of developing deep venous thrombosis versus not developing it among patients taking aspirin is roughly only half of the same odds among patients not taking aspirin.

A 95% CI for this overall OR is given by

$$\begin{aligned}
\ln \mathrm{OR}_{95\% \text{ CI}} &= \ln \mathrm{OR}_{\mathrm{Overall}} +/- 1.96 \times 1/\sqrt{\textstyle\sum w_i} \\
&= -0.731 +/- 1.96 \times 1/\sqrt{9.64} \\
&= -0.731 +/- 0.631 \\
&= (-1.362, -0.1).
\end{aligned}$$

Taking the inverse of the logarithm for both of these numbers yields

$$95\% \text{ CI}(0.26, 0.90).$$

The estimate of the overall OR can therefore be expressed as 0.48, 95% CI (0.26, 0.90). The inverse variance method is the simplest of the fixed effects meta-analysis methods. The other methods use very similar calculations.

8.8 Random Effects Methods

Random effects models take into consideration not only the amount of variance in each study but also the variance between studies. As noted, they are appropriate when there is significant heterogeneity. The DerSimonian and Laird method is the most popular random effects method for combining data from 2×2 tabes. Like the inverse variance method

$$\ln OR_{\text{DerSimonian and Laird (DL)}} = \frac{\sum w_{\text{DL}(i)} \ln OR_i}{\sum w_{\text{DL}(i)}}.$$

The difference is in how studies are weighted. The DerSimonian and Laird weighting for each study is given by

$$w_{\text{DL}(i)} = \frac{1}{\text{var}_i + \tau}.$$

The variance is calculated in the same way as the inverse variance method. "τ" is the Greek symbol "tau" and is given by

$$\tau = \frac{Q - (k - 1)}{\sum w_i - \frac{\sum(w_i^2)}{\sum w_i}},$$

where w_i is the same weight calculated according to the inverse variance method as $w_i = 1/\text{var}_i$, Q is Cochran's heterogeneity statistic, and k is the number of studies in the meta-analysis. If Q is less than $k - 1$, τ is assigned a value of 0, and $w_{\text{DL}(i)}$ is the same as it would be under the inverse variance method. This formula can be tedious. Rather than committing it to memory, it is more important for you to understand in general terms how random effects models take heterogeneity among studies into account.

8.9 Sensitivity Analysis

In the context of systematic reviews, sensitivity analysis refers to checking the robustness of conclusions by changing the way the systematic review is done. Consider the following example. A systematic review of a herbal remedy for migraines includes 10 studies and finds that the therapy is highly effective. Three of the studies, however, are of poorer quality than the other seven. The systematic reviewers decide to repeat their analysis, but this time by excluding the three lower quality studies. They still find that the therapy is highly effective. Their conclusion, therefore, has withstood one type of sensitivity analysis. Let us say that they pool data using a fixed effects model from all 10 studies together and find that the overall OR for relief of migraine with the herbal remedy compared to placebo is 6.0, 95% CI (4.0, 8.0). This is a highly significant result. To test the robustness of the conclusion that the herbal remedy is highly effective, they repeat the pooling of data using a random effects model. Since there is little statistical heterogeneity among the studies, they find that the overall

OR is 5.8, 95% CI (3.3, 8.3). The 95% CI is only slightly wider than with the fixed effects model. The systematic review has withstood another type of sensitivity analysis.

8.10 Bias in the Preparation of Systematic Reviews

Systematic reviews are prone to specific biases in the identification and selection of studies, which can dramatically influence their conclusions. The bias which has received the greatest attention is *publication bias*. Simply put, certain types of studies are more likely to published than others. A systematic review that incorporates only published studies, therefore, may have biased conclusions. In general, studies with statistically significant results are much more likely to be published than those without such results. A study of a new drug, for example, is more likely to be published if it shows that the drug is superior to an existing product. There are several reasons for this. Authors of studies are sometimes more likely to submit studies for publication if their results are positive. Pharmaceutical companies, which wield considerable influence over whether studies of their products are published, also encourage publication of significant studies and discourage publication of nonsignificant studies. Selective submission of studies is largely responsible for publication bias, though some journal editors may also be more likely to accept studies with significant findings. Publication bias can be reduced by making an effort to identify unpublished studies. Experts in a particular field can be contacted for their knowledge of any unpublished studies. There are also several "registries" of clinical trials. Investigators include details of trials in such registries that they plan to conduct prior to the availability of any results. Contacting investigators who have registered a relevant study but have not published any results is a worthwhile strategy for identifying unpublished studies.

Systematic reviews are also prone to other types of bias. Relevant studies for inclusion might be published but in a language other than English. A systematic review that incorporates only English language papers may miss important studies. It has been shown that English language papers are more likely to report positive findings than papers in other languages. This may be because investigators in non-English speaking countries are more likely to submit papers with significant results to international English language journals, and those with insignificant results to local journals. Searching only electronic databases for journal articles is also prone to bias. Many journals from developing countries, for example, are not indexed in Medline or Embase. Looking through the reference lists of relevant papers for additional studies in addition to electronic databases is valuable but is prone to *citation bias*—studies with positive findings are more likely to be cited than those with negative (insignificant) findings.

Systematic reviews are sometimes prone to bias in the provision of data. Let us say that you wish to complete a meta-analysis by pooling data from several 2 × 2 tables. You find that data required to complete some of the 2 × 2 tables is missing. In some cases, investigators whose studies revealed insignificant results may be more reluctant to provide necessary missing data than investigators whose studies revealed significant results.

Finally, systematic reviews are sometimes influenced by biased inclusion criteria. Systematic reviews are often prepared by investigators with extensive knowledge of the field. They may knowingly or unknowingly manipulate the inclusion criteria to include certain studies with which they are familiar or favor for some reason.

Although some of these biases are difficult or impossible to avoid, knowledge of them and a sincere effort to counteract their influence is an important part of the best way to prepare a systematic review. Efforts to identify unpublished or non-English language studies, for example, should be reported in a systematic review and suggest that it is of high quality.

8.11 Detecting Bias in Systematic Reviews

Publication bias and bias in locating studies such as English language bias or citation bias can be detected using a *funnel plot*. A funnel plot is simply a plot of the effect estimates of individual studies included in a systematic review against each study's sample size or a surrogate of the sample size. The idea behind a funnel plot is discussed next.

Larger studies yield more precise estimates of effect. Results from small studies yield more widely scattered effect estimates that may or may not show a benefit, for example, of a new therapy. Therefore, if effect size is plotted against sample size, the resulting plot should resemble a funnel *if there is no bias in the publication and identification of studies for the systematic review*. If the plot is asymmetrical or skewed in some way, bias may be present. The most common "abnormality" in a funnel plot is a gap in the wide part of the funnel, which suggests that a number of small studies that show no effect or even a harmful effect have either not been found or were not published.

Look carefully at Figure 8.4.

The plot uses the standard error of the log of the OR as a measure of precision and an indirect measure of sample size. (Larger studies are more precise and have a smaller standard error of log OR.) On the horizontal axis is the log OR. This is a funnel plot for a systematic review of a therapy

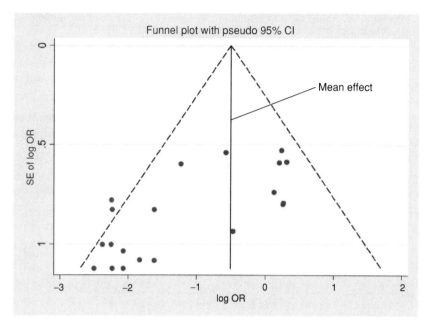

FIGURE 8.4 Sample Funnel Plot

(Reproduced from Bagshaw SM, Ghali WA. Acetylcysteine for prevention of contrast-induced nephropathy after intravascular angiography: A systematic review and meta-analysis. BMC Med 2004;2:38.)

designed to protect against an adverse event. Therefore, the smaller the log OR, the more protective is the therapy. Notice that there are several imprecise (small) studies scattered in the left lower corner of the funnel plot that show a substantial protective effect. There are fewer imprecise studies in the lower right portion of the plot. This is evidence, therefore, of publication bias.

Funnel plots are especially useful in the preparation of a systematic review. They can pinpoint the need for a search for additional studies. Alternatively, a sensitivity analysis can be performed with the exclusion of certain studies. At the very least, when bias is present, the conclusions of a systematic review should be tempered to reflect it. Often statements about bias are included with the results of a sensitivity analysis. You might have a statement in the conclusions of a systematic review like the following:

We found the new treatment to be highly effective. Through the use of a funnel plot however, we discovered significant bias. This likely represents publication bias, and the absence of several small studies with non-significant results. We decided to perform a sensitivity analysis that excludes all of the

smaller studies that showed a substantial beneficial effect from the review.
We still found the new treatment to be highly effective.

PROBLEMS

1. You are in the process of completing a systematic review to determine
    if breastfeeding during infancy is protective against childhood envi-
    ronmental allergies. You have found three, high-quality case-control
    studies and have assembled the following corresponding 2 × 2 tables
    (Tables 8.7–8.9).

TABLE 8.7   Study I

Breastfed	Environmental Allergies	
	+	−
+	14	86
−	21	79

TABLE 8.8   Study II

Breastfed	Environmental Allergies	
	+	−
+	6	194
−	8	192

TABLE 8.9   Study III

Breastfed	Environmental Allergies	
	+	−
+	26	174
−	28	172

How would you summarize the *individual* results of these three studies?

2. Assuming that heterogeneity of any kind is not a problem, calculate a
    summary, "pooled" summary result for the three studies.
3. How much inconsistency is present among the three studies?

SOLUTIONS TO PROBLEMS

1. The appropriate way to summarize the individual studies is with ORs. For study I, the OR is $14 \times 79/86 \times 21 = 0.61$. For study II, the OR is $6 \times 192/8 \times 194 = 0.74$. For study III, the OR is $26 \times 172/28 \times 174 = 0.92$.

   Ideally, since these studies were based on samples, these ORs should be accompanied by 95% CIs.

   For study I, the lower boundary of the 95% CI is given by

   $$\ln \text{OR}_{(\text{lower limit})} = \ln (0.61) - 1.96 \times \sqrt{1/14 + 1/79 + 1/86 + 1/21}$$
   $$= -1.24$$
   $$\text{OR}_{\text{lower limit}} = e^{-1.24} = 0.29.$$

   The upper limit is given by

   $$\ln \text{OR}_{(\text{upper limit})} = \ln (0.61) + 1.96 \times \sqrt{1 / 14 + 1/79 + 1/86 + 1/21}$$
   $$= 0.24$$
   $$\text{OR}_{\text{upper limit}} = e^{0.24} = 1.28.$$

   For study II, the lower boundary of the 95% CI is given by

   $$\ln \text{OR}_{(\text{lower limit})} = \ln (0.74) - 1.96 \times \sqrt{1/6 + 1/192 + 1/8 + 1/194}$$
   $$= -1.38$$
   $$\text{OR}_{\text{lower limit}} = e^{-1.38} = 0.25.$$

   The upper limit is given by

   $$\ln \text{OR}_{(\text{upper limit})} = \ln (0.74) + 1.96 \times \sqrt{1/6 + 1/192 + 1/8 + 1/194}$$
   $$= 0.78$$
   $$\text{OR}_{\text{upper limit}} = e^{0.78} = 2.17.$$

   For study III, the lower boundary of the 95% CI is given by

   $$\ln \text{OR}_{(\text{lower limit})} = \ln (0.92) - 1.96 \times \sqrt{1/26 + 1/172 + 1/28 + 1/174}$$
   $$= -0.66$$
   $$\text{OR}_{\text{lower limit}} = e^{-0.66} = 0.52.$$

TABLE 8.10   Summary of Results

Study	OR With 95% CI
I	0.61 (0.29, 1.29)
II	0.74 (0.25, 2.18)
III	0.92 (0.52, 1.63)

The upper boundary is given by

$$\ln OR_{(upper\ limit)} = \ln(0.92) + 1.96 \times \sqrt{1/26 + 1/172 + 1/28 + 1/174}$$
$$= 0.49$$
$$OR_{upper\ limit} = e^{0.49} = 1.63.$$

The results can therefore be summarized in Table 8.10.

2. If we can assume that heterogeneity of any kind (including statistical heterogeneity) is not an issue, one can use a fixed effects model to pool the data. The summary OR using the inverse variance method is given by

$$\ln OR_{Overall} = \frac{\sum w_i \ln OR_i}{\sum w_i}.$$

The weight of each study is given by the inverse of its variance. Recall that the variance of each study is given by

$$Var_i = \frac{1}{a_i} + \frac{1}{b_i} + \frac{1}{c_i} + \frac{1}{d_i}.$$

The variances and weights of each study are given next:

Study I. Var $= 1/14 + 1/79 + 1/86 + 1/21 = 0.14$; weight $= 1/0.14 = 7.0$.

Study II. Var $= 1/6 + 1/192 + 1/8 + 1/194 = 0.30$; weight $= 3.3$.

Study III. Var $= 1/26 + 1/172 + 1/28 + 1/174 = 0.086$; weight $= 11.7$.

The sum of these weights is $7.0 + 3.3 + 11.7 = 22.0$.
The sum of each weight multiplied by the natural log of each OR is

$$(7.0 \times \ln 0.67) + (3.3 \times \ln 0.74) + (11.7 \times \ln 0.92) = -4.77.$$

We can now calculate ln $OR_{Overall}$ as

$$-4.77/22 = -0.22$$
$$e^{-0.22} = 0.80.$$

This is the "overall" OR. The 95% CI is given by

$$\ln OR_{95\% \text{ CI}} = \ln OR_{Overall} \pm 1.96 \times 1/\sqrt{\sum w_i}$$
$$= -0.22 \pm 1.96 \times 1/\sqrt{22}$$
$$= -0.64, 0.20.$$
$$e^{-0.64} = 0.53; e^{0.20} = 1.22.$$

Our pooled estimate can therefore be summarized as OR = 0.80, 95% CI (0.53, 1.22).

3. To calculate inconsistency, we need Cochran's Q, which is given by

$$Q = \Sigma w_i [(\ln OR_i) - (\ln OR_{overall})]^2.$$

Fortunately we already have what we need to calculate Q. We need, $w_i [(\ln OR_i) - (\ln OR_{overall})]^2$ for each study.

For study I, this is 7.0 [(ln 0.61) − (ln 0.80)]^2 = 0.51.
For study II, 3.3[(ln 0.74) − (ln 0.80)]^2 = 0.02.
For study III, 11.7[(ln 0.92) − (ln0.80)]^2 = 13.5.

Q is therefore 0.22 + 0.02 + 13.5 = approximately 13.7.

Inconsistency can be measured as

$$I^2 = 100\% \times (Q - df)/Q.$$

For our three studies,

$$I^2 = 100\% \times (13.7 - 2)/13.7 = \text{approximately } 85\%.$$

There is therefore significant inconsistency among the three studies. We can conclude that 85% of the differences observed are not due to chance but to heterogeneity. Incidentally, a random effects model would have been more appropriate for obtaining the pooled OR. You were asked to assume no significant heterogeneity for Problem 2 for the sake of simplicity.

References

1. Sutton G. Putrid gums and "Dead Men's Cloaths": James Lind aboard the *Salisbury*. *J R Soc Med* 2003;96:605–608.
2. Rao G, Fisch L, Srinivasan S, D'Amico F, Okada T, Eaton C, et al. Does this patient have Parkinson disease? *JAMA* 2003;289(3):347–353.
3. Bagshaw SM, Ghali WA. Acetylcysteine for prevention of contrast-induced nephropathy after intravascular angiography: A systematic review and meta-analysis. *BMC Med* 2004;2:38.

Decision Analysis

OBJECTIVES

1. Define decision analysis.
2. Distinguish between the normative and descriptive perspectives of how humans make decisions.
3. List the steps involved in decision analysis.
4. Define utility.
5. Describe how the standard reference gamble can be used to calculate utility for different health states.
6. Combine life expectancies with utilities to calculate quality-adjusted life years.
7. List and describe the five axioms required for utility theory to be valid.
8. Given a decision problem and the necessary probabilities and utilities, construct a decision tree and use expected value decision making to determine the best course of action.
9. In general terms, describe how sensitivity analysis is applied to decision analyses.
10. Define cost-effectiveness.
11. In general terms, describe what is meant by a Markov process and a Monte Carlo simulation.
12. Provide an interpretation of a bubble diagram that depicts a Markov process.

9.1 Introduction

So far this book has addressed fairly straightforward questions. When comparing one diagnostic test to another, for example, we are interested in test that predicts the presence of a disease more accurately. In a study of two or more therapies, we are interested in therapy that is most effective. In reality, making rational medical decisions is more complicated. A new therapy for lung cancer, for example, may be more effective than an older therapy but may be associated with much worse side effects making its use intolerable. Despite their effectiveness, some therapies may be so expensive or inaccessible for other reasons that their use is not practical.

Rational medical decision making should not only address simple questions of effectiveness and accuracy but also a broader range of questions that take into consideration cost, availability, side effects, and patient preferences.

Decision analysis is a formal quantitative process that attempts to simulate human decision making by weighing the benefits and disadvantages of different options. The term decision analysis was coined in the 1960s. Decision analysis quickly became a popular strategy to compare different decision options in the business world. The use of decision analysis in healthcare is relatively new. The science of how humans should and do make decisions, however, has been around for nearly 300 years. There are three different perspectives or models for studies of how human beings make decisions about their health or many other aspects of life. The *normative* perspective assumes that people make rational choices based upon a few assumptions or *axioms*. One type of normative model will be discussed in detail later in this chapter. The *descriptive* perspective is based upon observations of how people actually make decisions in real life. Mathematical models based on this perspective are judged not based on how closely they match certain axioms but rather how closely they match the choices people actually make. The *prescriptive* perspective is based upon helping people make the best choices based upon descriptive and/or normative information. Through this perspective, strategies are compared and an optimal strategy is *prescribed*. Decision analysis is a prescriptive process with a normative foundation.

9.2 Process of Decision Analysis

Depending upon the problem and outcomes addressed and the precise techniques used, decision analysis can get very complicated. For most physicians what is important is having a basic understanding of what decision analysis is and how it works. The cases presented in this chapter are deliberately simplified. If interested in learning more, please consult the Annotated Bibliography.

Decision analysis can be broadly divided into four consecutive steps. First, one must precisely *define the problem being addressed*. This is not unlike defining a precise clinical question. Next, one must *structure the decision problem*. This is done using a *decision tree* which illustrates the options being considered and the potential outcomes of each option. The third *step is obtaining information necessary to solve the decision problem*. If you are trying to decide between two treatments for endometrial cancer, for example, you will need to know the probability of remission with each treatment. For decision analyses, such information is usually obtained from existing medical literature. Finally, one *chooses a preferred course of action* based on the structure of the decision problem and the information needed to solve it. Each of these four steps is illustrated in Case 9.1.

CASE 9.1

Mrs. Jarvis is a 60-year-old woman who faces an unfortunate situation. She has recently been diagnosed with a malignant brain tumor. She visits a neurosurgeon who recommends surgical removal of the tumor. She then visits an oncologist who recommends against surgery and tells her that a course of chemotherapy with radiation therapy is the best option. Finally, she visits a palliative care specialist who tells her that neither form of treatment is a good option and both are associated with a high level of risk and side effects with little chance of cure and long-term survival. He recommends palliation only. Mrs. Jarvis comes to you to ask what you think she should do. How would you characterize and structure this problem and what would you recommend?

The first step is to precisely characterize the decision problem. Mrs. Jarvis has to choose among three treatments. Let us assume for the time being that the only outcome she values is her life expectancy with each treatment. The decision problem is: *Among the options of surgery, chemotherapy + radiation therapy (medical therapy), and palliative care, which one is associated with the longest life expectancy in a patient with a malignant brain tumor?*

I told you that unlike straightforward studies of therapies and diagnostic tests, decision making using tools such as decision analyses takes many aspects of a healthcare decision into consideration. Case 9.1 has been simplified to illustrate some basic principles. In reality, most patients are not only interested in life expectancy but also in quality of life. Also, there may be more than three treatment options available. We will ignore these complexities for now. The second step is to structure the decision problem using a decision tree.

A decision tree is a graphical representation of the decision problem (Fig. 9.1). The decision to be made is represented by a square known as a *decision node*. Emanating from the decision node are lines that represent each decision option. In our case there are three options.

Each of these three options is associated with one or more outcomes. What could happen if Mrs. Jarvis has surgery? Well, the surgeon may successfully remove the tumor in which case she would live as long as she would have if she had no tumor in the first place. The surgery could go terribly wrong and Mrs. Jarvis could die on the operating table. In that case her life expectancy is effectively zero. Mrs. Jarvis could survive the surgery but the surgeon may not be able to extract the tumor. In that case she could die from natural progression of the disease. There is also the slim possibility that a miracle could take place and rather than dying of

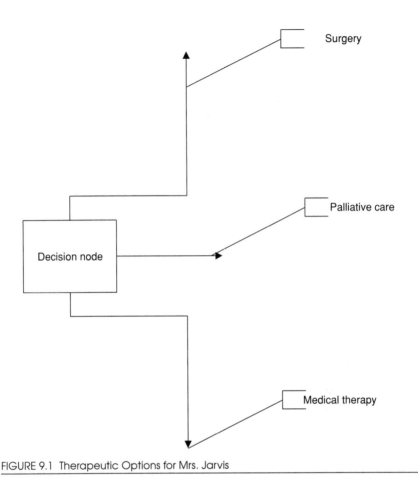

FIGURE 9.1 Therapeutic Options for Mrs. Jarvis

progression of the disease, Mrs. Jarvis could have a spontaneous cure despite an unsuccessful surgery. Let us limit our outcomes of surgery to
these four. In reality, there are many other possible outcomes. The surgeon
could remove part of the tumor, for example, and Mrs. Jarvis could have a
life expectancy in between that from natural progression of disease and a
cure. A greater number of outcomes adds to the complexity of the decision
problem.

What if Mrs. Jarvis chose the chemotherapy + radiation therapy (medical therapy) option? Medical therapy could be successful and Mrs. Jarvis
could be cured going on to fulfill her natural life expectancy. Medical therapy could also be completely unsuccessful and she could die from progression of disease. Let us limit our outcomes of medical therapy to these two.
In theory, the medical therapy could be unsuccessful and Mrs. Jarvis could
have a spontaneous cure. Let us assume that once Mrs. Jarvis receives

medical therapy, it is not possible to distinguish between a cure with medical therapy and a spontaneous cure.

Let us assume there are only two possible outcomes of palliative care. Mrs. Jarvis could either die of progression of disease (palliative care by definition is not curative). She could also have a miraculous spontaneous cure. We now have an inventory of possible outcomes to add to our decision tree. Each possible outcome emanates from a *chance node*, represented by a circle. Chance nodes are so named because there is a probability or chance associated with each outcome. Our decision tree now is given in Fig. 9.2.

Our decision tree provides our decision problem with structure. The next step is to obtain information necessary to solve the decision problem. We need to know, for example, what the probability of a cure of Mrs. Jarvis's brain tumor is with surgery. We also need to know what her life expectancy would be with different outcomes. Information about the probability of different outcomes is usually obtained from existing literature. This is often a difficult and time-consuming aspect of decision analysis. Obtaining an estimate of the probability of a single outcome, for example, may require doing a complete systematic review of literature that includes finding and evaluating studies that provide individual estimates of the probability. The decision analysis could then use a pooled estimate. The best estimate for each probability, however it is obtained, is called the *baseline* estimate. Most decision analyses use a range of estimates of probabilities of outcomes from the medical literature and solve the decision problem using different estimates of these probabilities. This process will be discussed in detail later in this chapter.

Life expectancies and other quantitative outcomes are also completed by reviewing existing literature. Life expectancy in some circumstances is fairly obvious. As noted, if Mrs. Jarvis died on the operating table, her life expectancy is essentially zero. If she is cured of the brain tumor and assuming she has no other illnesses, one can assume that she will live as long as the average woman, or roughly to the age of 80.

Let us assume that we have collected the information needed to solve our decision problem. We have three chance nodes and therefore need three sets of probabilities. Let us say we find that the probability of dying on the operating table during surgery for a brain tumor is roughly 5%. The probability of a cure is 70%. The probability of an unsuccessful surgery but with a spontaneous cure is 1%, and the probability of an unsuccessful surgery with disease progression is 24%. These probabilities represent all the possible outcomes of surgery. Notice that the sum of these four probabilities is 100% (or 1). *The sum of the probabilities at any chance node must add up to 1.* Otherwise, one or more outcomes having a chance of occurring has been excluded. With the palliative care option, let us assume that the probability of spontaneous cure is 5% and the probability of disease progression

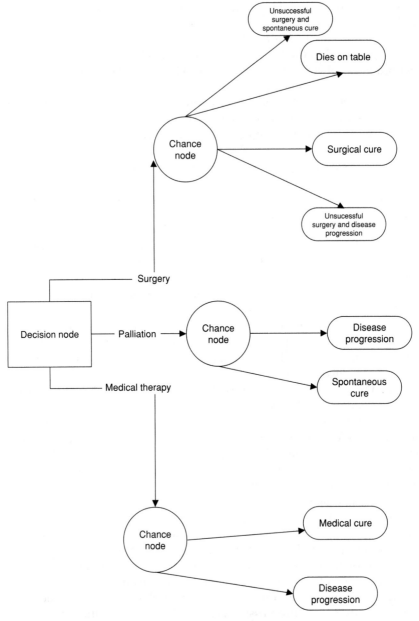

FIGURE 9.2 Decision Tree with Chance Nodes and Outcomes

is 95%. Notice that the probability of spontaneous cure with palliation is higher than that of unsuccessful surgery plus spontaneous cure, since the latter is the probability of two events occurring together. With the medical therapy option, let us assume that the chance of a cure is 66⅔% and that of disease progression is 33⅓%.

We now need estimates of life expectancies. As mentioned, if Mrs. Jarvis's brain tumor is cured she can expect to live to be about 80, or another 20 years. This is her life expectancy regardless of whether the cure is spontaneous or is the result of surgery or medical therapy. If she dies on the table her life expectancy is zero. If her disease progresses, regardless of which type of treatment she receives, let us assume she can expect to live about 2 years. We now have all the information needed to solve our decision problem. Figure 9.3 shows the decision tree with the probabilities and life expectancies included.

Solving the decision problem means determining which one is best for the patient. In this case, since Mrs. Jarvis wants to live as long as possible, we wish to determine the option which we expect would yield the highest life expectancy *on the average*. This process is known as *expected value decision making*. The calculations involved are quite simple. We calculate the expected value of life expectancy with each treatment option. To do this, we start at the ends of our decision tree and multiply each probability at each chance node by its life expectancy and add up the resulting values at each chance node to obtain the expected value of life expectancy with each treatment. This process is known as *folding back*.

Some decision trees have more that one chance node associated with each treatment option. As we have depicted them, there are two distinct unsuccessful surgery outcomes with a total probability of occurring of 0.25: unsuccessful surgery with disease progression and unsuccessful surgery with spontaneous cure. Our decision tree could have included a broad outcome of unsuccessful surgery from which emanates a chance node with these two more specific outcomes, each with a specific probability (see Fig. 9.4). In such circumstances, one multiplies the probability of each of these more specific outcomes by its associated life expectancy and adds up these values for the chance node. Then, this total life expectancy associated with the chance node is multiplied by the probability of the broader outcome (unsuccessful surgery) to obtain the total expected value of life expectancy for the treatment in question (unsuccessful surgery in this case).

Let us fold back the simple decision tree in Fig. 9.2. The expected value associated with the option of surgery is the following:

Expected value of surgery = p(unsuccessful + spontaneous cure) × 20 + p(dies on table) × 0 + p(surgical cure) × 20 + p(unsuccessful + disease

progression) × 2 = (0.01 × 20) + (0.05 × 0) + (0.70 × 20) + (0.24 × 2)

= 14.68 years.

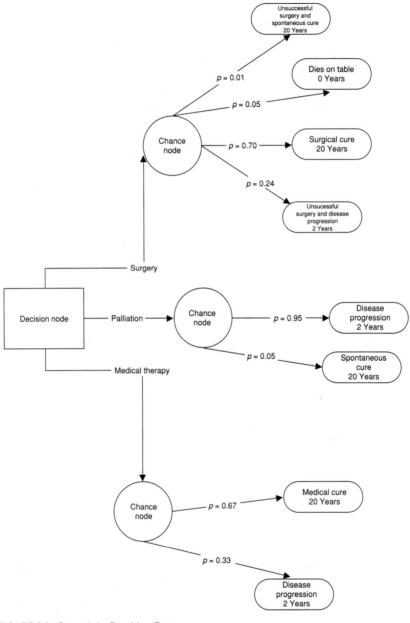

FIGURE 9.3 Complete Decision Tree

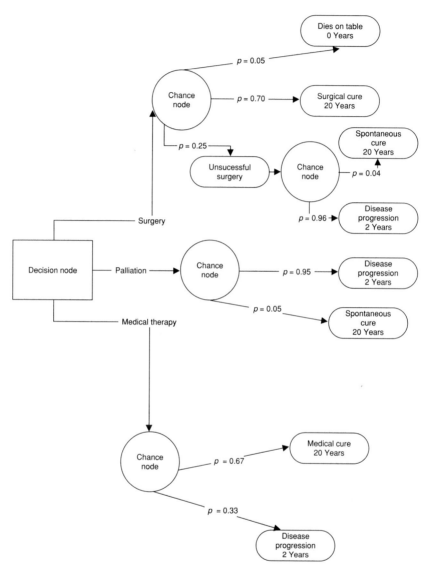

FIGURE 9.4 Decision Tree with Chance Node Associated with Outcome of Unsuccessful Surgery

The expected value of palliative care is the following:

Expected value of palliative care $= (0.95 \times 2) + (0.05 \times 20) = 2.9$ years.

The expected value of medical therapy is the following:

Expected value of medical therapy $= (0.67 \times 20) + (0.33 \times 2) = 14.06$ years.

The expected value of surgery is highest, even though the difference between the surgical and medical options is small. Based on expected value decision making, therefore, we can conclude that Mrs. Jarvis should choose the option of surgery.

9.3 Utility

The example of expected value decision making presented in the previous section is not only simple, but also somewhat unrealistic. It is unlikely that any patient would care only about life expectancy as an outcome. Imagine that one possible outcome of surgery was complete paralysis but with a normal life expectancy of 20 years. Taking only life expectancy into account ignores *quality of life*. The outcomes of different treatment strategies can be expressed not only in terms of life expectancy but also as quality of life measures. *Utility* is one such measure and can be defined as the strength of a person's preference for different outcomes. Utility is measured on a scale of 0 to 1 where 1 usually represents the best possible outcome that could result by following one or more of the strategies described in a decision analysis. For Case 9.1, for example, the best possible outcome is cure of the brain tumor with a life expectancy of 20 years. This outcome can be assigned a utility of 1. Death is often the worst possible outcome of a treatment strategy and is usually assigned a utility of 0. (There are some exceptional circumstances that are worse than death to many people.) The utility of any outcomes other than death and the best possible outcome must be assigned a utility between 0 and 1.

There are many ways to determine the utility associated with different health states. A group of experts may reach a consensus about the utility of a particular health state based on their clinical experience. Such a group could, for example, conclude that the utility of paralysis of both lower limbs after neurological surgery is 0.6, meaning that it is much better than death, but not nearly as good as a state of "full health." Previously published medical literature is also a rich source of data on utilities for a number of different health states. Such data is collected systematically from patients through surveys and interviews. One approach to determining the utility of specific health states to individual patients was first described by von Neumann and Morganstern in 1944[1] and makes use of what is known as the *standard reference gamble*, an example of which is given in Case 9.2.

CASE 9.2

Mrs. Jarvis is no longer only concerned with the life expectancy associated with different treatments for her brain tumor. One possible outcome of surgery is complete blindness, an outcome she would of course like to avoid. Her preferred outcome remains cure of her brain tumor with a normal life expectancy. Her least preferred outcome is death. How can you help to determine the utility of complete blindness to Mrs. Jarvis?

First, we can assign a utility of 0 to death and 1 to cure of the tumor with normal life expectancy. To determine the utility of complete blindness we set up a standard reference gamble. In a standard reference gamble, an individual is faced with the choice between an outcome with intermediate utility, which is a sure thing, and a gamble for the best and worst possible outcomes. An appropriate standard reference gamble for Mrs. Jarvis might resemble the following:

Mrs. Jarvis, I want you to consider the following situation. Assume that you are completely blind. I have a bag of 10 balls. The balls are either red or white, but you have no way of telling which color each is when you select one. The bag must have at least one ball of each color. If you select a white ball, your sight will be restored. If you select a red ball, you will die. What is the maximum number of red balls you are willing to tolerate in the bag before you choose to participate in this gamble?

Let us say that Mrs. Jarvis says that she would tolerate only two red balls (and therefore eight white balls) in the bag before blindly selecting a ball. What does this mean? It means that she does not wish to take more than a 20% chance of drawing a red ball and dying for the chance of restoring her sight. Intuitively you can imagine that for Mrs. Jarvis, blindness is not such a bad state of health. Let us say I have another patient who faces Mrs. Jarvis's situation but when presented with the gamble, tells you that he is willing to tolerate a maximum of eight red balls in the bag. This tells you that blindness is a terrible state for him and he is desperate for even a 20% chance of restoring his sight despite the 80% risk of death. One can conclude that the utility of blindness is higher for Mrs. Jarvis than for the second patient. More specifically we can calculate the utility (U) of any intermediate state with the following equation:

$$U_{[\text{intermediate state}]} = p_{[\text{indifference}]} \times U_{[\text{best state}]} + (1 - p_{[\text{indifference}]}) \times U_{[\text{worst state}]},$$

where $p_{[\text{indifference}]}$ stands for "indifference probability"—the probability at which the subject is "indifferent" between the sure thing and the gamble. In Mrs. Jarvis's case, for example, if there were fewer than eight white balls in the bag, there is no question that she would not participate in the gamble. Similarly, if there were nine white balls in the bag, there is no question that she would participate in the gamble. The indifference probability is the "threshold" point of eight white balls, which represents a $p_{[indifference]}$ of 0.8. The utility of blindness is therefore

$$U_{[blindness]} = 0.8 \times 1 + 0.2 \times 0 = 0.8.$$

We have therefore solved for the unknown utility of blindness using the utilities of two known states, full sight and death.

Just as we used life expectancy, we can use utilities as the outcomes in decision trees. Utilities are clearly more versatile since they can apply to a range of treatments that do not affect life expectancy and take quality of life into account. Utilities can also be combined with life expectancies to calculate *quality-adjusted life years* (QALYs). Let us say that one outcome of a particular treatment for cancer is chronic fatigue but a normal life expectancy of approximately 30 years after treatment. A standard reference gamble has revealed that the utility of living with chronic fatigue is 0.7. We calculate QALYs in the following way:

$$30 \text{ years} \times 0.7 = 21 \text{ QALYs.}$$

QALYs can also be used to describe outcomes in which the utility changes with time. Let us say that for one outcome, the total life expectancy is 20 years. The first 5 years have a utility of 1 and the next 10 years have a utility of 0.5. The outcome can be described as

$$5 \text{ years} \times 1 + 10 \text{ years} \times 0.5 = 10 \text{ QALYs.}$$

9.4 Axioms for Determining Utility Using a Standard Reference Gamble

Utility theory depends upon five important axioms or conditions that must be met in order for it to be valid:

1. Given any two outcomes of a gamble, the participant in the gamble must be able to express a preference for one of them. For example, if there was a gamble in which possible outcomes were blindness and complete paralysis, the participant must have a preference for one or the other. His strength of preference for both outcomes cannot be identical.

2. Preferences must always be *transitive*. This means that if an outcome A is preferred to another B, which in turn is preferred to C, then A must be preferred to C.

3. If A is preferred to B and B is preferred to C, there must be an indifference probability associated with B as a "sure thing."

4. If A is preferred to B, the participant in the gamble must choose the situation which gives him the highest chance of winning A. (This axiom should seem obvious.)

5. All gambles that involve the same probability of winning the same prizes (preferred outcome states) are equivalent, regardless of whether the prizes are won in one drawing or several drawings occurring at the same time. In other words, a single gamble in which a participant has a 20% chance of winning a preferred prize is equivalent to multiple simultaneous gambles in which the probability of winning the same prize is also 20%.

9.5 Sensitivity Analysis

We discussed sensitivity analysis with respect to systematic reviews, whereby the robustness of conclusions of a systematic review are tested by excluding the results of certain studies and repeating the analysis. Decision analysis employs a similar process. A decision tree is repeatedly folded back using different values for probabilities and utilities (or life expectancies). Often, estimates of probability, for example, are associated with a margin of error or imprecision. For Case 9.1, we might have a surgical cure rate of 70% (0.70) estimated from the literature. Such a cure rate might be associated with a margin of error expressed as a 95% CI:

$$\text{Surgical cure rate} = 0.70, 95\% \text{ CI } (0.60, 0.80).$$

We could perform a sensitivity analysis by folding back the tree and calculating the expected value of the surgery option using the lower boundary of this CI (0.60) and then repeating our calculation of the expected value by using the upper boundary of the CI (0.80). Let us consider the lower boundary estimate. Since the probability of all events at each chance node must add up to 1, the probability of the other potential outcomes may change when we use 0.60 as the surgical cure rate. Let us say that the other outcome probabilities assume the following values:

$p[\text{unsuccessful} + \text{spontaneous cure}] = 0.01$

$p[\text{dies on table}] = 0.05$

$p[\text{unsuccessful} + \text{disease progression}] = 0.34$

The only value that has changed is the probability of unsuccessful surgery with disease progression.

The expected value of the surgery option becomes

Expected value of surgery $= (0.01 \times 20) + (0.05 \times 0) + (0.60 \times 20)$
$$+ (0.34 \times 2) = 12.88 \text{ years.}$$

Notice that this falls well below our previously calculated value for the expected value of medical therapy. We cannot be so confident that surgery is the superior option. Sensitivity analysis, as you can imagine, can get very complicated. In many decision analyses, there is a range of estimates associated with each probability. Utility estimates can also vary tremendously. There is also the whole matter of using different estimates in combination. For example, if the estimate for the probability of a medical cure was given as 0.67, 95% CI (0.60, 0.74), we could use the lower boundary of the CI for medical cure and the lower boundary of the CI for the surgery option and then recalculate the expected values to determine which treatment is superior. The number of possible combinations of estimates in a single decision tree is very large. It is reasonable to use different values for probabilities and utilities only for estimates which are especially uncertain (e.g., come from poor quality studies).

Sensitivity analysis in which only one estimate is varied at a time is known as *one-way sensitivity analysis*. The results of such a sensitivity analysis can be expressed using a graph as shown in Fig. 9.5.

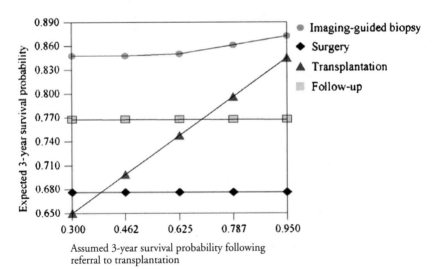

FIGURE 9.5 Impact of Varying Estimate of Initial 3-Year Survival Upon Expected 3-Year Survival

(*Reproduced with permission from El-Serag H, Mallat DB, Rabeneck L. Management of the single liver nodule in a cirrhotic patient. A decision analysis model. J Clin Gastroenterol 2005;39:157.*)

This graph comes from a decision analysis developed to decide how to treat liver nodules appearing in patients with liver cirrhosis.[2] Four treatment options, including liver transplantation, are represented by the different lines. The probability that is varied is the estimated 3-year survival of patients when they are first referred to a clinic for possible transplantation. The expected 3-year survival probability is the outcome that is being measured. One can conclude that as the initial assumed 3-year survival probability changes, there is no change in the expected value for survival for the treatment options of surgery and routine follow-up. The expected value of 3-year survival increases slightly with imaging-guided biopsy as higher estimates are used for the assumed initial 3-year survival probability. Notice the dramatic impact of varying initial assumed 3-year survival probability upon the treatment effect of transplantation. Notice also that depending upon the assumed 3-year survival probability, transplantation is either "better" or "worse" than the options of "surgery" and "follow-up."

9.6 Cost-Effectiveness Analysis

Consumers of the medical literature are likely to encounter variations of decision analysis that incorporate two other methods: cost-effectiveness analysis and Markov processes. As in the case of decision analysis in general, the procedures can get very complicated. What is presented here are a few basic principles that will help you understand these approaches.

To this point, we have discussed what is best for individual patients. In the case of Mrs. Jarvis, for example, we tried to maximize her life expectancy. Health care systems and increasingly, health care providers, have a responsibility not only to provide optimal care for individual patients but also to allocate resources in the most rational way that maximizes benefit for all patients. *Cost-effectiveness analysis* is a comparison of different strategies in terms of their cost per unit of output. Cost-effectiveness analysis is often incorporated into decision analysis, as illustrated in Case 9.3.

CASE 9.3

Your patient Alice, age 52, has recently been diagnosed with advanced hepatitis C disease. She faces three treatment alternatives: liver transplantation (which carries a significant risk of death), interferon therapy, and a conservative approach that includes only treatment of complications, abstinence from alcohol and other hepatotoxic agents, and good nutrition. A decision tree with life expectancy (LE) as the principal outcome is shown in Fig. 9.6.

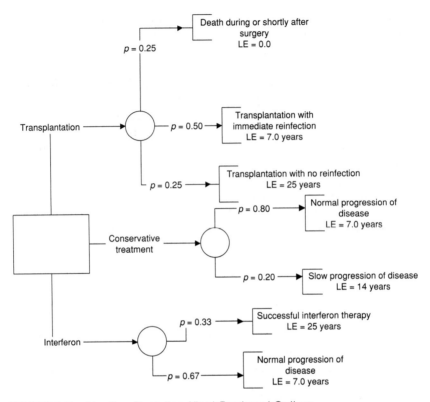

FIGURE 9.6 Decision Tree Depicting Alice's Treatment Options

The life-time costs associated with each of the treatments are the following:

Transplantation $200,000

Interferon $400,000

Conservative Treatment $60,000

Let's complete a simple cost-effectiveness analysis using the information provided.

We start by folding back our decision tree to calculate the expected
value of life expectancy for the three different treatments. For surgery, expected value of life expectancy is

$$0.0 \times 0.25 + 7.0 \times 0.50 + 25 \times 0.25 = 9.75 \text{ years.}$$

For interferon therapy, expected value of life expectancy is

$$25 \times 0.33 + 7.0 \times 0.67 = 12.94 \text{ years.}$$

For conservative treatment, expected value of life expectancy is

$$7.0 \times 0.80 + 14 \times 0.20 = 8.4 \text{ years.}$$

Based upon life expectancy, interferon therapy is best on the average. However, it is also the most expensive treatment. We can calculate the cost per year of life for each treatment:

Transplantation—$200,000/9.75 years = $20,513 per year

Interferon—$400,000/12.94 years = $30,913 per year

Conservative treatment—$60,000/8.4 years = $7,142 per year

Years of life cost less with conservative treatment than with the other treatments. This does not necessarily mean that this is the best treatment option. After all, if we were only interested in saving money, we would do nothing (total cost $0.00) and Alice would probably survive for 7 years.

It may be more reasonable to compare the two other options in terms of cost. We use the general formula for cost effectiveness:

$$\text{Cost effectiveness} = \frac{\text{costs with A} - \text{costs with B}}{\text{outcome with A} - \text{outcome with B}}.$$

For interferon versus transplantation,

$$\text{Cost effectiveness} = \frac{\$400,000 - \$200,000}{12.94 \text{ years} - 9.75 \text{ years}} = \$62,696/\text{extra year.}$$

The "cost" per unit of "effect" is more than $62,696 per year. Physicians, insurance companies, hospitals, etc. use this type of information to determine if such a cost is worth the extra life expectancy based on the resources they have and the need to provide services for other patients.

9.7 Markov Processes

Conventional decision trees such as those we have discussed so far in this chapter describe how a person in one state of health could wind up in another over a fixed period of time. In Mrs. Jarvis's case, for example, if she has surgery, she winds up in one of four states of health, which, for the sake of simplicity she reaches almost immediately. This is not the usual situation with many chronic disease processes. For certain cancers, for example, it is possible to obtain a remission with therapy, followed by a period of good health, and then a relapse of cancer, and then eventually death. Conventional decision trees do not do a good job of accounting for changes in states of health over a long period of time. A *Markov process* describes the transitions of a group of patients from one state of health to another. Instead of considering transitions over a fixed or short time period, Markov processes describe transitions over series of short intervals known as cycles. In each cycle, a patient has a probability of changing from one health state to another. These probabilities can change with time. Markov processes are often depicted with *bubble diagrams* such as the one shown in Fig. 9.7.[3]

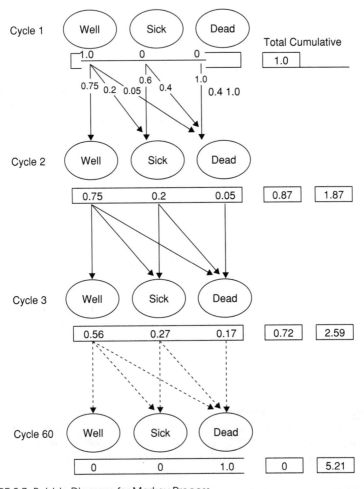

FIGURE 9.7 Bubble Diagram for Markov Process

(Reproduced with permission from Naimark D, Krahn MD, Naglie G, Redelmeier DA, Detsky AS. Primer on medical decision analysis: Part 5—Working with Markov processes. Med Decis Making 1997;17:153.)

This simple bubble diagram does not depict any specific disease process. There are three potential health states. Each cycle represents a time interval (e.g., 1 month). The numbers just below each oval represent the proportion of the cohort of patients that is in each state. At the beginning (Cycle 1), therefore, all patients are well. The numbers in the arrows below the first-cycle ovals are *transition probabilities*—the probability of moving from one state to another. For instance, if a patient is well in Cycle 1, he/she has a 0.75 probability of remaining well and a 0.2 probability of becoming sick in Cycle 2. Notice that some probabilities are impossible. It is not possible with many progressive chronic diseases to go from being sick to well, and always impossible to go from death to any other state. Death is known as an *absorbing state*, since that is the state in which all patients will eventually wind up. The fundamental feature of a Markov process is that the distribution of future states depends only upon the present state and not on how patients got to the present state. For example, the distribution of states in Cycle 3 depends only upon the distribution of states in Cycle 2 and the transition probabilities.

"Total" indicates the total utility of patients in that cycle. In Cycle 1, for example, all patients are well and the total utility is therefore 1. In this example, the utility of "sick" happens to be 0.6, and of course, the utility of death is 0. "Cumulative" indicates the sum of total utilities across cycles. After 60 cycles, all patients have died. The total utility is 5.21. It is not possible to have any more cycles since all patients have entered the absorbing state.

Markov processes may seem a bit obscure and, needless to say, are unfamiliar to most physicians. One way to make things more clear is to describe a Markov process using what is called a *Monte Carlo simulation*. Consider the natural course of a patient infected with hepatitis C. Let us say I have a jar with 100 colored balls. The jar contains 90 white balls that represent remaining in an asymptomatic state. The jar also contains 10 red balls that represent becoming ill with hepatitis C. The probability of transitioning from the asymptomatic to the ill state is therefore 0.10 or 10%. Without looking, you draw a ball from the jar. If it is white, your patient remains asymptomatic. If it is red, your patient becomes ill. You draw a white ball from the jar and then return it to the jar. On four subsequent drawings you draw white balls, each time replacing the drawn ball to the jar. On the next drawing, you draw a red ball. Your patient has now entered the ill state. Each drawing represents one cycle in the Markov process. Each cycle could represent a time period of 1 month or 1 year. This entire process of drawing balls until a red one is selected is repeated 99 times for a total of 100 times. The average number of white balls drawn each time represents the average time that a patient remains asymptomatic before becoming ill. Now that the patient has entered the ill state, a second jar is filled with

100 balls. Ninety of these are red and represent remaining ill. Ten are black and represent dying from complications of liver disease. Once again, you draw balls in succession until you draw a black ball and your patient enters the absorbing state. This process is also repeated over and over again to determine the average length of life in the ill state before death. Monte Carlo simulations are normally performed by computers given the large number of calculations involved.

You will find papers that use Markov processes to model the natural course of disease, or the course of disease with different approaches. Markov processes are sometimes indicated as parts of decision trees with a *Markov node*, which looks like a chance node but contains a symbol for "infinity" (∞).

Sources that contain more advanced information about Markov processes can be found in the Annotated Bibliography.

PROBLEMS

1. Stan is a 50-year-old man who suffers from chronic low back pain secondary to a herniated vertebral disc. He is presented with three treatment options. He could have surgery for the disc. This is associated with a 60% chance of complete relief of symptoms (utility = 1.0), 35% chance of continued low back pain symptoms of the same severity (utility = 0.5), and a 5% chance of death (utility = 0.0). He could have steroid injections for the pain. This option is associated with a 50% chance of complete relief of symptoms (utility = 1.0), a 25% chance of partial relief of symptoms (utility = 0.75), and a 25% chance of continued low back pain symptoms of the same severity (utility = 0.5). Stan could also choose medication therapy. This option is associated with a 10% chance of complete relief of symptoms (utility = 1.0), a 30% chance of partial relief of symptoms (utility = 0.75), and a 60% chance of continued symptoms nearly of the same severity (utility = 0.6). Construct a decision tree and calculate the expected value of utility for the three different treatment options.

2. The actual estimate of the utility of continued symptoms falls within a range of 0.40–0.60. How, if at all, does this change what you would recommend for Stan?

3. The cost of surgery (with follow-up care, etc.) is $25,000. The cost of periodic steroid injections over the course of the remainder of Stan's life is $27,500. What is the cost-effectiveness of steroid injections? (Use the values of utility you calculated in Problem 1.)

4. You are helping your patient Marcello prepare a "living will" whereby he discusses his wishes for end-of-life care and life-sustaining

treatment if he falls gravely ill. One of the questions that come up during this discussion is how he feels about losing his sense of smell, a condition known as "anosmia." You set up a standard reference gamble with 10 imaginary balls in a bag. White balls represent restoration of his normal sense of smell. Black balls represent death. You ask Marcello what is the maximum number of black balls he is willing to tolerate in the bag assuming that there must be at least one ball of each color. He tells you that there is no way he would participate in the gamble. What can you conclude about the utility of anosmia for Marcello? In what type of gamble may Marcello be more willing to participate?

SOLUTIONS TO PROBLEMS

1. The decision tree is shown in Fig. 9.8.
    The expected values of utility for the different treatment options are the following:

    Surgery—Expected $U = 0 \times 0.05 + 1.0 \times 0.60 + 0.50 \times 0.35 = 0.78$.

    Steroid injections—Expected $U = 1.0 \times 0.50 + 0.75 \times 0.25 + 0.50 \times 0.25 = 0.81$.

    Medications: Expected $U = 1.0 \times 0.10 + 0.75 \times 0.30 + 0.50 \times 0.60 = 0.63$.

    Steroid injections yield a slightly higher expected utility than surgery and should be the preferred option based on the information provided.

2. Let us assume that the utility of continued symptoms falls at the lower boundary of the range (0.40). Our expected utilities become:

    Surgery—Expected $U = 0 \times 0.05 + 1.0 \times 0.60 + 0.40 \times 0.35 = 0.74$

    Steroid injections—Expected $U = 1.0 \times 0.50 + 0.75 \times 0.25 + 0.40 \times 0.25 = 0.79$

    Medications—Expected $U = 1.0 \times 0.10 + 0.75 \times 0.30 + 0.40 \times 0.60 = 0.57$

    Now let us assume that the utility of continued symptoms falls at the higher boundary of the range (0.60). Our expected utilities become:

    Surgery—Expected $U = 0 \times 0.05 + 1.0 \times 0.60 + 0.60 \times 0.35 = 0.81$

    Steroid injections—Expected $U = 1.0 \times 0.50 + 0.75 \times 0.25 + 0.60 \times 0.25 = 0.84$

    Medications—Expected $U = 1.0 \times 0.10 + 0.75 \times 0.30 + 0.60 \times 0.60 = 0.69$

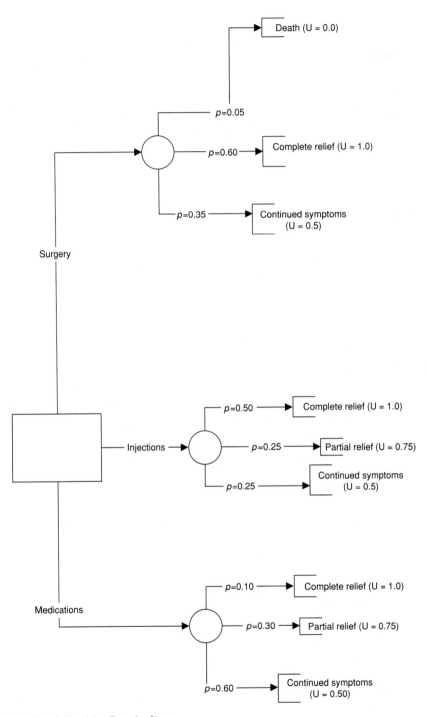

FIGURE 9.8 Decision Tree for Stan

This one-way sensitivity analysis does not change our conclusion that steroid injections are a slightly superior option to surgery for Stan.

3. $\text{Cost-effectiveness} = \dfrac{\text{costs with A} - \text{costs with B}}{\text{outcome with A} - \text{outcome with B}}.$

   In this situation, $\text{Cost-effectiveness} = \dfrac{\$27{,}500 - \$25{,}000}{0.81 - 0.78} = \$83{,}333$

$$\text{per unit of utility.}$$

This is a very high cost per unit of utility. Most people would conclude that the extra cost of steroid injections is not worth the slightly higher utility.

4. Marcello does not want to participate in the gamble because he is unwilling to accept even a 10% chance of drawing a black "death" ball to restore his sense of smell. His indifference probability, the probability at which he is indifferent between the sure thing (i.e., not being able to smell) and participating in the gamble, is therefore less than 10%.
   Let us assume for a moment that he is willing to accept one black ball before choosing to participate. His utility of anosmia would be

$$U_{[anosmia]} = 0.90 \times 1.0 + 0.10 \times 0 = 0.9$$

Since he is actually unwilling to accept a 10% chance of drawing a black ball, meaning that the chance of drawing a white ball would have to be higher than 0.90, his utility of anosmia is >0.90. Marcello may be willing to participate in a gamble in which the probability of drawing a black ball is significantly less than 0.10. Suppose we have a bag not with 10 balls but with 100 balls. We could then ask Marcello about the maximum number of black balls he is willing to tolerate among the bag of 100 white and black balls. If he says he is willing to tolerate only one black ball, we can calculate his utility of anosmia as the following:

$$U_{[anosmia]} = 0.99 \times 1.0 + 0.01 \times 0 = 0.99.$$

References

1. von Neumann J, Morganstern O. *Theory of Games and Economic Behavior.* Princeton, NJ: Princeton University Press; 1944.
2. El-Serag H, Mallat D, Rabeneck L. Management of the single liver nodule in a cirrhotic patient: A decision analysis model. *J Clin Gastroenterol* 2005;39(2):152–159.
3. Naimark D, Krahn MD, Naglie G, Redelmeier DA, Detsky AS. Primer on decision analysis: Part 5—Working with Markov processes. *Med Decis Making* 1997;17:152–159.

Clinical Practice Guidelines

10

1. Define clinical practice guideline (CPG) and describe the rationale for development of CPGs.
2. Describe the structured format for summary of CPGs from the National Guideline Clearinghouse.
3. Distinguish between the strength of a practice recommendation and the quality of evidence supporting a recommendation.
4. Describe how the US Preventive Services Task Force classifies the strength of recommendations and quality of evidence.
5. In general terms, describe the Delphi method for reaching consensus.

10.1 Introduction

A clinical practice guideline (CPG) is a systematically developed statement that includes recommendations, policies, or algorithms for the care of patients with specific problems or risks. A CPG on type 2 diabetes, for example, may include recommendations for screening, diagnosis, medication therapy, etc. More commonly, CPGs do not encompass all aspects of a particular disease but rather address a few specific questions. For example, there are a number of guidelines that describe the diagnostic criteria for diabetes and do not address issues of therapy. However, CPGs are distinct from systematic reviews and other forms of research papers in that they rarely address only one specific clinical question. Rather than pooling evidence together, the goal of CPGs is to develop one or more recommendations based on evidence in its final form. Development of CPGs involves the skill of critical appraisal as well as formal methods of developing consensus among panels of experts. CPGs are also distinct from systematic reviews and other types of research papers in that they rarely deal with only one, straightforward outcome. A systematic review of the effectiveness of one type of medication for heart failure, for example, may conclude that the medication should be used in all patients. The medication may, however, be too expensive to be used for all patients. It may be associated with side effects so serious that its widespread use is impossible. Such factors are normally taken into consideration as the recommendations that make up a CPG are assembled.

10.2 Rationale

The ultimate purpose of CPGs is to serve as a vehicle for "putting research into practice." Imagine that a new research study finds that potassium supplementation significantly lowers blood pressure among patients with hypertension. Ideally, based on this finding, physicians around the world ought to recommend potassium supplementation for their hypertensive patients. Unfortunately, most physicians do not have the time or the inclination to absorb all relevant research papers in their original form. "Summary services," which summarize relevant research papers to make them easier to digest, are used by some physicians. In addition to providing summaries (similar to abstracts), some of these services provide recommendations on how to apply the research findings in practice. A summary of one research paper, however, cannot take into consideration all the other factors (e.g., cost, patient comfort, availability of treatments, etc.) that make up rational medical decision making. A CPG about treatment of hypertension, however, can incorporate a recommendation of potassium supplementation along with other recommendations about treatment. If followed carefully, a CPG allows physicians to help their patients' benefit from the best available evidence from recent research. CPGs are developed for one or more of the following reasons:

- To improve the quality of care
- To improve cost-effectiveness
- To serve as educational tools

10.3 Description of CPGs

Federal organizations, health insurers, professional specialty organizations, and others publish CPGs as freestanding papers or in medical journals. The Internet has become an important means of disseminating CPGs. Indeed, the National Guideline Clearinghouse (NGC), a service of the Agency for Health Care Research and Quality (AHRQ), has among the largest, most comprehensive, and easy-to-use collections of CPGs currently available (see www.guideline.gov). The NGC uses a structured format for CPGs. Guideline developers are encouraged to follow this format. Missing elements may indicate a weakness in the methodology used to develop a guideline. In addition to basic information about the source, funding, availability, and category of problem addressed, the NGC summary format includes several important categories of information that all guideline developers should supply:

1. Scope. The scope of a guideline includes the specific circumstances in which it should be used. This means the disease or condition to which it applies, the intended users (e.g., primary care physicians, specialists), the objectives of the guideline (e.g., to save money, decrease unnecessary and harmful diagnostic testing, etc.), the patients to whom the guideline applies, the interventions being considered, and the major outcomes being considered (e.g., admission rate to hospital).

2. Methodology. Guideline developers should provide a description of the methods used to search for, select, and analyze evidence. They should also describe explicitly how the evidence was used to formulate recommendations. In some cases, a guideline may have been *validated*, meaning that its impact upon clinical practice has been assessed, it has been evaluated by independent reviewers, or it has been formally compared to other guidelines addressing the same problem. The results of such a validation should be described in the methodology.

3. Recommendations. Guideline developers should describe the major recommendations of the guideline. Often, these are provided in the form of an algorithm.

4. Evidence supporting recommendations. Each recommendation should be accompanied by a description of the evidence supporting it.

5. Benefits/harms of implementing the recommendations: Anticipated potential benefits and harms of implementing the guideline should be described.

6. Contraindications. In some special circumstances, use of a CPG may be inappropriate. These "contraindications" should be included in a summary.

7. Qualifying statements. A qualifying statement is a "disclaimer" or a statement of caution about how the guideline should be interpreted. Not all guidelines, of course, include the qualifying statement. A summary of a guideline entitled *Endoscopic retrograde cholangiopancreatography (a diagnostic technique for liver and related diseases) for diagnosis and therapy*, for example, included the qualifying statement:

> *The statement reflects the panel's assessment of medical knowledge available at the time the statement was written. Thus, it provides a "snapshot in time" of the state of knowledge on the conference topic. When reading the statement, keep in mind that new knowledge is inevitably accumulating through medical research.*[1]

8. Implementation of the guideline. This is a description of strategies used to promote use of the guideline and measurement of the impact of the guideline in practice.

10.4 Classification of Recommendations

One common source of confusion among consumers of CPGs is the way in which practice recommendations are characterized. The *strength* of a recommendation refers to whether there is enough quality evidence to support or not support it. The *quality of evidence* behind a particular recommendation refers to the methodological rigor of one or more studies that address the recommendation. Strength of recommendations and quality of evidence are, as you might imagine, usually, congruent: the better the quality of evidence, the stronger is a specific recommendation. There are several similar rating systems for strength of recommendations and quality of evidence. The scheme used by the US Preventive Services Task Force (USPSTF), which develops and disseminates many guidelines for screening and prevention, is widely used.[2]

The U.S. Preventive Services Task Force (USPSTF) grades its recommendations according to one of five classifications (A, B, C, D, I) reflecting the strength of evidence and magnitude of net benefit (benefits minus harms).

    A.— *The USPSTF strongly recommends that clinicians provide [the service] to eligible patients. The USPSTF found good evidence that [the service] improves important health outcomes and concludes that benefits substantially outweigh harms.*

    B.— *The USPSTF recommends that clinicians provide [this service] to eligible patients. The USPSTF found at least fair evidence that [the service] improves important health outcomes and concludes that benefits outweigh harms.*

    C.— *The USPSTF makes no recommendation for or against routine provision of [the service]. The USPSTF found at least fair evidence that [the service] can improve health outcomes but concludes that the balance of benefits and harms is too close to justify a general recommendation.*

    D.— *The USPSTF recommends against routinely providing [the service] to asymptomatic patients. The USPSTF found at least fair evidence that [the service] is ineffective or that harms outweigh benefits.*

    I.— *The USPSTF concludes that the evidence is insufficient to recommend for or against routinely providing [the service]. Evidence that the [service] is effective is lacking, of poor quality, or conflicting and the balance of benefits and harms cannot be determined. The USPSTF grades the* *quality of the overall evidence for a service on a 3-point scale (good, fair, poor):*

Good: *Evidence includes consistent results from well-designed, well-conducted studies in representative populations that directly assess effects on health outcomes.*

Fair: *Evidence is sufficient to determine effects on health outcomes, but the strength of the evidence is limited by the number, quality, or consistency of the individual studies, generalizability to routine practice, or indirect nature of the evidence on health outcomes.*

Poor: *Evidence is insufficient to assess the effects on health outcomes because of limited number or power of studies, important flaws in their design or conduct, gaps in the chain of evidence, or lack of information on important health outcomes.*

A typical "A" recommendation is "The USPSTF strongly recommends that clinicians screen all adults for tobacco use and provide tobacco cessation interventions for those who use tobacco products."[3]

The evidence behind the recommendation was described as "The USPSTF found good quality evidence examining the efficacy of various levels of intensity of tobacco cessation counseling by clinicians based on a meta-analysis of 43 studies."[3]

10.5 Reaching Consensus

Ideally, high-quality evidence would be available to support practice recommendations in every guideline. Under such circumstances, guideline development would involve nothing more than extracting evidence from original research papers from which practice recommendations would naturally follow. Unfortunately, it is rare that good evidence is available for all important decisions that make up a practice guideline. Moreover, interpretation and application of good evidence, even when available, is always somewhat subjective. The majority of CPGs therefore rely at least to some extent upon a "consensus" (agreement among a group) of individuals, who are usually experts in the field addressed by the guideline, or experts in partnership with other stakeholders such as health care insurers, patients, etc. There are many ways in which consensus is reached in the development of guidelines. Some guidelines are assembled without a careful examination of evidence, and based only upon the opinions of a small group of individuals presented at one meeting. Such guidelines are especially prone to the biases of the participating guideline developers. In some groups, the opinions of one or two individuals may dominate and the resulting guideline is unlikely to represent a balance of opinions at the meeting. The majority of guidelines depend at least to some extent upon reaching a consensus among individuals. Indeed, you will find that many practice guidelines include the terms, *consensus statement* or *consensus development conference* in their titles. The *Delphi* method is among the most popular ways to reach consensus. The Delphi method was developed by the scientists from the Research and Development (RAND) corporation in the 1940s. RAND researchers argued that in fields that had not developed to the point of having well-established scientific laws, it was permissible to use the testimony of experts. This circumstance is analogous to that which many guideline developers face today: Expert opinion is used to fill the gaps where evidence is lacking. The Delphi method relies upon communication among a group of experts who may or may not be in the same place. A series of questionnaires is sent to the group to elicit responses to very specific problems. Responses to each questionnaire are analyzed and subsequent questionnaires reflect this analysis. Participants are given feedback about responses from the group at different stages in the process. All participants remain anonymous. This facilitates more candid responses from group members. The Delphi method can get complicated but here is a simple example that will give you the general idea: Imagine a group of experts that has been asked to decide which antibiotics are best to prescribe for ear infections in children. Group members are asked through mailed questionnaires to list their three preferred antibiotics. Each first choice antibiotic is assigned 3 points, second choice antibiotics are assigned 2 points, and third choice antibiotics are assigned 1 point. The responses are compiled, and the total points participants assigned to different antibiotics are shared with the group. In a second questionnaire, only the three antibiotics receiving the highest scores from the first questionnaire are listed as options, and participants are asked to indicate their first, second, and third preference. Once again, this information is compiled and analyzed and the information is shared with the group. A third questionnaire could be sent to participants, which includes only the two antibiotics from the second questionnaire that received the highest points. Participants could be asked to indicate their preference for one of the two.

Anonymous mailed surveys of the type described before are often combined with live "consensus" meetings. For example, if the number of participants selecting each of the antibiotics in a third survey as described in the previous example was roughly equal, a live meeting could be held to openly discuss differences of opinion with the aim of reaching some sort of consensus. Such live meetings are especially helpful when experts do not interpret questionnaires in the same way. It is possible, for example, that some experts are basing their choice of "best antibiotic" on which one is most likely to prevent serious complications, while others are concerned with which one is associated with fewer side effects.

10.6 Implementation of CPGs

Ultimately, the success of a practice guideline depends upon whether physicians are willing and able to implement it in practice. Implementation remains a huge problem. In the late 1990s, the US Agency for Health Care Research and Quality invested an enormous amount of time and money in developing high-quality, evidence-based practice guidelines only to find a few years later that they had had little impact upon clinical practice. Strategies to implement the recommendations in guidelines are as crucial as the recommendations themselves. Changing physicians' behavior to comply with new practice guidelines is a major challenge. Physicians sometimes view practice guidelines as inflexible and a threat to their autonomy. The success of a practice guideline depends upon strategies such as using physician leaders in a practice, hospital, or community to communicate the recommendations, and establishing a system of reminders of recommendations whenever a patient to whom the guideline applies is being seen.

References

1. Agency for Health Care Research and Quality (AHRQ). National guideline clearinghouse. URL: www.guideline.gov. Accessed 20 October, 2005.
2. Harris RP, Helfand M, Woolf SH, Lohr KN, Mulrow CD, Teutsch SM, Atkins D. Current methods of the U.S. Preventive Services Task Force: A review of the process. *Am J Prev Med* 2001;20(suppl 3):21–35.
3. U.S. Preventive Services Task Force. Counseling: Tobacco use. URL: www.ahrq.gov/clinic/uspstf/uspstbac.htm. Accessed December 31, 2005.

Appendix

TABLE A.1 Normal Distribution

(a)

Probability content from $-\infty$ to z

z	0.00	0.01	0.02	0.03	0.04	0.05	0.06	0.07	0.08	0.09
0.0	0.5000	0.5040	0.5080	0.5120	0.5160	0.5199	0.5239	0.5279	0.5319	0.5359
0.1	0.5398	0.5438	0.5478	0.5517	0.5557	0.5596	0.5636	0.5675	0.5714	0.5753
0.2	0.5793	0.5832	0.5871	0.5910	0.5948	0.5987	0.6026	0.6064	0.6103	0.6141
0.3	0.6179	0.6217	0.6255	0.6293	0.6331	0.6368	0.6406	0.6443	0.6480	0.6517
0.4	0.6554	0.6591	0.6628	0.6664	0.6700	0.6736	0.6772	0.6808	0.6844	06879
0.5	0.6915	0.6950	0.6985	0.7019	0.7054	0.7088	0.7123	0.7157	0.7190	0.7224
0.6	0.7257	0.7291	0.7324	0.7357	0.7389	0.7422	0.7454	0.7486	0.7517	0.7549
0.7	0.7580	0.7611	0.7642	0.7673	0.7704	0.7734	0.7764	0.7794	0.7823	0.7852
0.8	0.7881	0.7910	0.7939	0.7967	0.7995	0.8023	0.8051	0.8078	0.8106	0.8133
0.9	0.8159	0.8186	0.8212	0.8238	0.8264	0.8289	0.8315	0.8340	0.8365	0.8389
1.0	0.8413	0.8438	0.8461	0.8485	0.8508	0.8531	0.8554	0.8577	0.8599	0.8621
1.1	0.8643	0.8665	0.8686	0.8708	0.8729	0.8749	0.8770	0.8790	0.8810	0.8830
1.2	0.8849	0.8869	0.8888	0.8907	0.8925	0.8944	0.8962	0.8980	0.8997	0.9015
1.3	0.9032	0.9049	0.9066	0.9082	0.9099	0.9115	0.9131	0.9147	0.9162	0.9177
1.4	0.9192	0.9207	0.9222	0.9236	0.9251	0.9265	0.9279	0.9292	0.9306	0.9319

z									
1.5	0.9332	0.9345	0.9357	0.9370	0.9382	0.9394	0.9406	0.9418	0.9429	0.9441
1.6	0.9452	0.9463	0.9474	0.9484	0.9495	0.9505	0.9515	0.9525	0.9535	0.9545
1.7	0.9554	0.9564	0.9573	0.9582	0.9591	0.9599	0.9608	0.9616	0.9625	0.9633
1.8	0.9641	0.9649	0.9656	0.9664	0.9671	0.9678	0.9686	0.9693	0.9699	0.9706
1.9	0.9713	0.9719	0.9726	0.9732	0.9738	0.9744	0.9750	0.9756	0.9761	0.9767
2.0	0.9772	0.9778	0.9783	0.9788	0.9793	0.9798	0.9803	0.9808	0.9812	0.9817
2.1	0.9821	0.9826	0.9830	0.9834	0.9838	0.9842	0.9846	0.9850	0.9854	0.9857
2.2	0.9861	0.9864	0.9868	0.9871	0.9875	0.9878	0.9881	0.9884	0.9887	0.9890
2.3	0.9893	0.9896	0.9898	0.9901	0.9904	0.9906	0.9909	0.9911	0.9913	0.9916
2.4	0.9918	0.9920	0.9922	0.9925	0.9927	0.9929	0.9931	0.9932	0.9934	0.9936
2.5	0.9938	0.9940	0.9941	0.9943	0.9945	0.9946	0.9948	0.9949	0.9951	0.9952
2.6	0.9953	0.9955	0.9956	0.9957	0.9959	0.9960	0.9961	0.9962	0.9963	0.9964
2.7	0.9965	0.9966	0.9967	0.9968	0.9969	0.9970	0.9971	0.9972	0.9973	0.9974
2.8	0.9974	0.9975	0.9976	0.9977	0.9977	0.9978	0.9979	0.9979	0.9980	0.9981
2.9	0.9981	0.9982	0.9982	0.9983	0.9984	0.9984	0.9985	0.9985	0.9986	0.9986
3.0	0.9987	0.9987	0.9987	0.9988	0.9988	0.9989	0.9989	0.9989	0.9990	0.9990

(continued)

TABLE A.1   Normal Distribution (*Continued*)

(b)

Far right tail probabilities

z	P{Z to ∞}	z	P{Z to ∞}	z	P{Z to ∞}
2.0	0.02275	3.0	0.001350	4.0	0.00003167
2.1	0.01786	3.1	0.0009676	4.1	0.00002066
2.2	0.01390	3.2	0.0006871	4.2	0.00001335
2.3	0.01072	3.3	0.0004834	4.3	0.00000854
2.4	0.00820	3.4	0.0003369	4.4	0.000005413
2.5	0.00621	3.5	0.0002326	4.5	0.000003398
2.6	0.004661	3.6	0.0001591	4.6	0.000002112
2.7	0.003467	3.7	0.0001078	4.7	0.000001300
2.8	0.002555	3.8	0.00007235	4.8	7.933 E-7
2.9	0.001866	3.9	0.00004810	4.9	4.792 E-7

z	P{Z to ∞}
5.0	2.867 E-7
5.5	1.899 E-8
6.0	9.866 E-10
6.5	4.016 E-11
7.0	1.280 E-12
7.5	3.191 E-14
8.0	6.221 E-16
8.5	9.480 E-18
9.0	1.129 E-19
9.5	1.049 E-21

This table is in public domain and produced by APL programs written by the author William Knight.

TABLE A.2   Critical Values of F Corresponding to $p<.05$ and $p<.01$

ν_n

ν_d	1	2	3	4	5	6	7	8	9	10	11	12	14	16	20	24	30	40	50	75	100	200	500	x
1	161	200	216	225	230	234	237	239	241	242	243	244	245	246	248	249	250	251	252	253	253	254	254	254
	4052	**4999**	**5403**	**5625**	**5764**	**5859**	**5928**	**5981**	**6022**	**6056**	**6082**	**6106**	**6142**	**6169**	**6208**	**6234**	**6261**	**6286**	**6302**	**6323**	**6334**	**6352**	**6361**	**6366**
2	18.51	19.00	19.16	19.25	19.30	19.33	19.36	19.37	19.38	19.39	19.40	19.41	19.42	19.43	19.44	19.45	19.46	19.47	19.47	19.48	19.49	19.49	19.50	19.50
	98.49	**99.00**	**99.17**	**99.25**	**99.30**	**99.33**	**99.36**	**99.37**	**99.39**	**99.40**	**99.41**	**99.42**	**99.43**	**99.44**	**99.45**	**99.46**	**99.47**	**99.48**	**99.48**	**99.49**	**99.49**	**99.49**	**99.50**	**99.50**
3	10.13	9.55	9.28	9.12	9.01	8.94	8.88	8.84	8.81	8.78	8.76	8.74	8.71	8.69	8.66	8.64	8.62	8.60	8.58	8.57	8.56	8.54	8.54	8.53
	34.12	**30.82**	**29.46**	**28.71**	**28.24**	**27.91**	**27.67**	**27.49**	**27.34**	**27.23**	**27.13**	**27.05**	**26.92**	**26.83**	**26.69**	**26.60**	**26.50**	**26.41**	**26.35**	**26.27**	**26.23**	**26.18**	**26.14**	**26.12**
4	7.71	6.94	6.59	6.39	6.26	6.16	6.09	6.04	6.00	5.96	5.93	5.91	5.87	5.84	5.80	5.77	5.74	5.71	5.70	5.68	5.66	5.65	5.64	5.63
	21.20	**18.00**	**16.69**	**15.98**	**15.52**	**15.21**	**14.98**	**14.80**	**14.66**	**14.54**	**14.45**	**14.37**	**14.24**	**14.15**	**14.02**	**13.93**	**13.83**	**13.74**	**13.69**	**13.61**	**13.57**	**13.52**	**13.48**	**13.46**
5	6.61	5.79	5.41	5.19	5.05	4.95	4.88	4.82	4.78	4.74	4.70	4.68	4.64	4.60	4.56	4.53	4.50	4.46	4.44	4.42	4.40	4.38	4.37	4.36
	16.26	**13.27**	**12.06**	**11.39**	**10.97**	**10.67**	**10.45**	**10.29**	**10.15**	**10.05**	**9.96**	**9.89**	**9.77**	**9.68**	**9.55**	**9.47**	**9.38**	**9.29**	**9.24**	**9.17**	**9.13**	**9.07**	**9.04**	**9.02**
6	5.99	5.14	4.76	4.53	4.39	4.28	4.21	4.15	4.10	4.06	4.03	4.00	3.96	3.92	3.87	3.84	3.81	3.77	3.75	3.72	3.71	3.69	3.68	3.67
	13.74	**10.92**	**9.78**	**9.15**	**8.75**	**8.47**	**8.26**	**8.10**	**7.98**	**7.87**	**7.79**	**7.72**	**7.60**	**7.52**	**7.39**	**7.31**	**7.23**	**7.14**	**7.09**	**7.02**	**6.99**	**6.94**	**6.90**	**6.88**
7	5.59	4.74	4.35	4.12	3.97	3.87	3.79	3.73	3.68	3.63	3.60	3.57	3.52	3.49	3.44	3.41	3.38	3.34	3.32	3.29	3.28	3.25	3.24	3.23
	12.25	**9.55**	**8.45**	**7.85**	**7.46**	**7.19**	**7.00**	**6.84**	**6.71**	**6.62**	**6.54**	**6.47**	**6.35**	**6.27**	**6.15**	**6.07**	**5.98**	**5.90**	**5.85**	**5.78**	**5.75**	**5.70**	**5.67**	**5.65**
8	5.32	4.46	4.07	3.84	3.69	3.58	3.50	3.44	3.39	3.34	3.31	3.28	3.23	3.20	3.15	3.12	3.08	3.05	3.03	3.00	2.98	2.96	2.94	2.93
	11.26	**8.65**	**7.59**	**7.01**	**6.63**	**6.37**	**6.19**	**6.03**	**5.91**	**5.82**	**5.74**	**5.67**	**5.56**	**5.48**	**5.36**	**5.28**	**5.20**	**5.11**	**5.06**	**5.00**	**4.96**	**4.91**	**4.88**	**4.86**
9	5.12	4.26	3.86	3.63	3.48	3.37	3.29	3.23	3.18	3.13	3.10	3.07	3.02	2.98	2.93	2.90	2.86	2.82	2.80	2.77	2.76	2.73	2.72	2.71
	10.56	**8.02**	**6.99**	**6.42**	**6.06**	**5.80**	**5.62**	**5.47**	**5.35**	**5.26**	**5.18**	**5.11**	**5.00**	**4.92**	**4.80**	**4.73**	**4.64**	**4.56**	**4.51**	**4.45**	**4.41**	**4.36**	**4.33**	**4.31**
10	4.96	4.10	3.71	3.48	3.33	3.22	3.14	3.07	3.02	2.97	2.94	2.91	2.86	2.82	2.77	2.74	2.70	2.67	2.64	2.61	2.59	2.56	2.55	2.54
	10.04	**7.56**	**6.55**	**5.99**	**5.64**	**5.39**	**5.21**	**5.06**	**4.95**	**4.85**	**4.78**	**4.71**	**4.60**	**4.52**	**4.41**	**4.33**	**4.25**	**4.17**	**4.12**	**4.05**	**4.01**	**3.96**	**3.93**	**3.91**
11	4.84	3.98	3.59	3.36	3.20	3.09	3.01	2.95	2.90	2.86	2.82	2.79	2.74	2.70	2.65	2.61	2.57	2.53	2.50	2.47	2.45	2.42	2.41	2.40
	9.65	**7.20**	**6.22**	**5.67**	**5.32**	**5.07**	**4.88**	**4.74**	**4.63**	**4.54**	**4.46**	**4.40**	**4.29**	**4.21**	**4.10**	**4.02**	**3.94**	**3.86**	**3.80**	**3.74**	**3.70**	**3.66**	**3.62**	**3.60**
12	4.75	3.88	3.49	3.26	3.11	3.00	2.92	2.85	2.80	2.76	2.72	2.69	2.64	2.60	2.54	2.50	2.46	2.42	2.40	2.36	2.35	2.32	2.31	2.30
	9.33	**6.93**	**5.95**	**5.41**	**5.06**	**4.82**	**4.65**	**4.50**	**4.39**	**4.30**	**4.22**	**4.16**	**4.05**	**3.98**	**3.86**	**3.78**	**3.70**	**3.61**	**3.56**	**3.49**	**3.46**	**3.41**	**3.38**	**3.36**

(continued)

TABLE A.2 Critical Values of F Corresponding to $p < .05$ and $p < .01$ (Continued)

ν_n

ν_d	1	2	3	4	5	6	7	8	9	10	11	12	14	16	20	24	30	40	50	75	100	200	500	x
13	4.67 **9.07**	3.80 **6.70**	3.41 **5.74**	3.18 **5.20**	3.02 **4.86**	2.92 **4.62**	2.84 **4.44**	2.77 **4.30**	2.72 **4.19**	2.67 **4.10**	2.63 **4.02**	2.60 **3.96**	2.55 **3.85**	2.51 **3.78**	2.46 **3.67**	2.42 **3.59**	2.38 **3.51**	2.34 **3.42**	2.32 **3.37**	2.28 **3.30**	2.26 **3.27**	2.24 **3.21**	2.22 **3.18**	2.21 **3.16**
14	4.60 **8.86**	3.74 **6.51**	3.34 **5.56**	3.11 **5.03**	2.96 **4.69**	2.85 **4.46**	2.77 **4.28**	2.70 **4.14**	2.65 **4.03**	2.60 **3.94**	2.56 **3.86**	2.53 **3.80**	2.48 **3.70**	2.44 **3.62**	2.39 **3.51**	2.35 **3.43**	2.31 **3.34**	2.27 **3.26**	2.24 **3.21**	2.21 **3.14**	2.19 **3.11**	2.16 **3.06**	2.14 **3.02**	2.13 **3.00**
15	4.54 **8.68**	3.68 **6.36**	3.29 **5.42**	3.06 **4.89**	2.90 **4.56**	2.79 **4.32**	2.70 **4.14**	2.64 **4.00**	2.59 **3.89**	2.55 **3.80**	2.51 **3.73**	2.48 **3.67**	2.43 **3.56**	2.39 **3.48**	2.33 **3.36**	2.29 **3.29**	2.25 **3.20**	2.21 **3.12**	2.18 **3.07**	2.15 **3.00**	2.12 **2.97**	2.10 **2.92**	2.08 **2.89**	2.07 **2.87**
16	4.49 **8.53**	3.63 **6.23**	3.24 **5.29**	3.01 **4.77**	2.85 **4.44**	2.74 **4.20**	2.66 **4.03**	2.59 **3.89**	2.54 **3.78**	2.49 **3.69**	2.45 **3.61**	2.42 **3.55**	2.37 **3.45**	2.33 **3.37**	2.28 **3.25**	2.24 **3.18**	2.20 **3.10**	2.16 **3.01**	2.13 **2.96**	2.09 **2.98**	2.07 **2.86**	2.04 **2.80**	2.02 **2.77**	2.01 **2.75**
17	4.45 **8.40**	3.59 **6.11**	3.20 **5.18**	2.96 **4.67**	2.81 **4.34**	2.70 **4.10**	2.62 **3.93**	2.55 **3.79**	2.50 **3.68**	2.45 **3.59**	2.41 **3.52**	2.38 **3.45**	2.33 **3.35**	2.29 **3.27**	2.23 **3.16**	2.19 **3.08**	2.15 **3.00**	2.11 **2.92**	2.08 **2.86**	2.04 **2.79**	2.02 **2.76**	1.99 **2.70**	1.97 **2.67**	1.96 **2.65**
18	4.41 **8.28**	3.55 **6.01**	3.16 **5.09**	2.93 **4.58**	2.77 **4.25**	2.66 **4.01**	2.58 **3.85**	2.51 **3.71**	2.46 **3.60**	2.41 **3.51**	2.37 **3.44**	2.34 **3.37**	2.29 **3.27**	2.25 **3.19**	2.19 **3.07**	2.15 **3.00**	2.11 **2.91**	2.07 **2.83**	2.04 **2.78**	2.00 **2.71**	1.98 **2.68**	1.95 **2.62**	1.93 **2.59**	1.92 **2.57**
19	4.38 **8.18**	3.52 **5.93**	3.13 **5.01**	2.90 **4.50**	2.74 **4.17**	2.63 **3.94**	2.55 **3.77**	2.48 **3.63**	2.43 **3.52**	2.38 **3.43**	2.34 **3.36**	2.31 **3.30**	2.26 **3.19**	2.21 **3.12**	2.15 **3.00**	2.11 **2.92**	2.07 **2.84**	2.02 **2.76**	2.00 **2.70**	1.96 **2.63**	1.94 **2.60**	1.91 **2.54**	1.90 **2.51**	1.88 **2.49**
20	4.35 **8.10**	3.49 **5.85**	3.10 **4.94**	2.87 **4.43**	2.71 **4.10**	2.60 **3.87**	2.52 **3.71**	2.45 **3.56**	2.40 **3.45**	2.35 **3.37**	2.31 **3.30**	2.28 **3.23**	2.23 **3.13**	2.18 **3.05**	2.12 **2.94**	2.08 **2.86**	2.04 **2.77**	1.99 **2.69**	1.96 **2.63**	1.92 **2.56**	1.90 **2.53**	1.87 **2.47**	1.85 **2.44**	1.84 **2.42**
21	4.32 **8.02**	3.47 **5.78**	3.07 **4.87**	2.84 **4.37**	2.68 **4.04**	2.57 **3.81**	2.49 **3.65**	2.42 **3.51**	2.37 **3.40**	2.32 **3.31**	2.28 **3.24**	2.25 **3.17**	2.20 **3.07**	2.15 **2.99**	2.09 **2.88**	2.05 **2.80**	2.00 **2.72**	1.96 **2.63**	1.93 **2.58**	1.89 **2.51**	1.87 **2.47**	1.84 **2.42**	1.82 **2.38**	1.81 **2.36**
22	4.30 **7.94**	3.44 **5.72**	3.05 **4.82**	2.82 **4.31**	2.66 **3.99**	2.55 **3.76**	2.47 **3.59**	2.40 **3.45**	2.35 **3.35**	2.30 **3.26**	2.26 **3.18**	2.23 **3.12**	2.18 **3.02**	2.13 **2.94**	2.07 **2.83**	2.03 **2.75**	1.98 **2.67**	1.93 **2.58**	1.91 **2.53**	1.87 **2.46**	1.84 **2.42**	1.81 **2.37**	1.80 **2.33**	1.78 **2.31**
23	4.28 **7.88**	3.42 **5.66**	3.03 **4.76**	2.80 **4.26**	2.64 **3.94**	2.53 **3.71**	2.45 **3.54**	2.38 **3.41**	2.32 **3.30**	2.28 **3.21**	2.24 **3.14**	2.20 **3.07**	2.14 **2.97**	2.10 **2.89**	2.04 **2.78**	2.00 **2.70**	1.96 **2.62**	1.91 **2.53**	1.88 **2.48**	1.84 **2.41**	1.82 **2.37**	1.79 **2.32**	1.77 **2.28**	1.76 **2.26**
24	4.26 **7.82**	3.40 **5.61**	3.01 **4.72**	2.78 **4.22**	2.62 **3.90**	2.51 **3.67**	2.43 **3.50**	2.36 **3.36**	2.30 **3.25**	2.26 **3.17**	2.22 **3.09**	2.18 **3.03**	2.13 **2.93**	2.09 **2.85**	2.02 **2.74**	1.98 **2.66**	1.94 **2.58**	1.89 **2.49**	1.86 **2.44**	1.82 **2.36**	1.80 **2.33**	1.76 **2.27**	1.74 **2.23**	1.73 **2.21**

df																								
25	4.24 **7.77**	3.38 **5.57**	2.99 **4.68**	2.76 **4.18**	2.60 **3.86**	2.49 **3.63**	2.41 **3.46**	2.34 **3.32**	2.28 **3.21**	2.24 **3.13**	2.20 **3.05**	2.16 **2.99**	2.11 **2.89**	2.06 **2.81**	2.00 **2.70**	1.96 **2.62**	1.92 **2.54**	1.87 **2.45**	1.84 **2.40**	1.80 **2.32**	1.77 **2.29**	1.74 **2.23**	1.72 **2.19**	1.71 **2.17**
26	4.22 **7.72**	3.37 **5.53**	2.98 **4.64**	2.74 **4.14**	2.59 **3.82**	2.47 **3.59**	2.39 **3.42**	2.32 **3.29**	2.27 **3.17**	2.22 **3.09**	2.18 **3.02**	2.15 **2.96**	2.10 **2.86**	2.05 **2.77**	1.99 **2.66**	1.95 **2.58**	1.90 **2.50**	1.85 **2.41**	1.82 **2.36**	1.78 **2.28**	1.76 **2.25**	1.72 **2.19**	1.70 **2.15**	1.69 **2.13**
27	4.21 **7.68**	3.35 **5.49**	2.96 **4.60**	2.73 **4.11**	2.57 **3.79**	2.46 **3.56**	2.37 **3.39**	2.30 **3.26**	2.25 **3.14**	2.20 **3.06**	2.16 **2.98**	2.13 **2.93**	2.08 **2.83**	2.03 **2.74**	1.97 **2.63**	1.93 **2.55**	1.88 **2.47**	1.84 **2.38**	1.80 **2.33**	1.76 **2.25**	1.74 **2.21**	1.71 **2.16**	1.68 **2.12**	1.67 **2.10**
28	4.20 **7.64**	3.34 **5.45**	2.95 **4.57**	2.71 **4.07**	2.56 **3.76**	2.44 **3.53**	2.36 **3.36**	2.29 **3.23**	2.24 **3.11**	2.19 **3.03**	2.15 **2.95**	2.12 **2.90**	2.06 **2.80**	2.02 **2.71**	1.96 **2.60**	1.91 **2.52**	1.87 **2.44**	1.81 **2.35**	1.78 **2.30**	1.75 **2.22**	1.72 **2.18**	1.69 **2.13**	1.67 **2.09**	1.65 **2.06**
29	4.18 **7.60**	3.33 **5.42**	2.93 **4.54**	2.70 **4.04**	2.54 **3.73**	2.43 **3.50**	2.35 **3.33**	2.28 **3.20**	2.22 **3.08**	2.18 **3.00**	2.14 **2.92**	2.10 **2.87**	2.05 **2.77**	2.00 **2.68**	1.94 **2.57**	1.90 **2.49**	1.85 **2.41**	1.80 **2.32**	1.77 **2.27**	1.73 **2.19**	1.71 **2.15**	1.68 **2.10**	1.65 **2.06**	1.64 **2.03**
30	4.17 **7.56**	3.32 **5.39**	2.92 **4.51**	2.69 **4.02**	2.53 **3.70**	2.42 **3.47**	2.34 **3.30**	2.27 **3.17**	2.21 **3.06**	2.16 **2.98**	2.12 **2.90**	2.09 **2.84**	2.04 **2.74**	1.99 **2.66**	1.93 **2.55**	1.89 **2.47**	1.84 **2.38**	1.79 **2.29**	1.76 **2.24**	1.72 **2.16**	1.69 **2.13**	1.66 **2.07**	1.64 **2.03**	1.62 **2.01**
32	4.15 **7.50**	3.30 **5.34**	2.90 **4.46**	2.67 **3.97**	2.51 **3.66**	2.40 **3.42**	2.32 **3.25**	2.25 **3.12**	2.19 **3.01**	2.14 **2.94**	2.10 **2.86**	2.07 **2.80**	2.02 **2.70**	1.97 **2.62**	1.91 **2.51**	1.86 **2.42**	1.82 **2.34**	1.76 **2.25**	1.74 **2.20**	1.69 **2.12**	1.67 **2.08**	1.64 **2.02**	1.61 **1.98**	1.59 **1.96**
34	4.13 **7.44**	3.28 **5.29**	2.88 **4.42**	2.65 **3.93**	2.49 **3.61**	2.38 **3.38**	2.30 **3.21**	2.23 **3.08**	2.17 **2.97**	2.12 **2.89**	2.08 **2.82**	2.05 **2.76**	2.00 **2.66**	1.95 **2.58**	1.89 **2.47**	1.84 **2.38**	1.80 **2.30**	1.74 **2.21**	1.71 **2.15**	1.67 **2.08**	1.64 **2.04**	1.61 **1.98**	1.59 **1.94**	1.57 **1.91**
36	4.11 **7.39**	3.26 **5.25**	2.86 **4.38**	2.63 **3.89**	2.48 **3.58**	2.36 **3.35**	2.28 **3.18**	2.21 **3.04**	2.15 **2.94**	2.10 **2.86**	2.06 **2.78**	2.03 **2.72**	1.98 **2.62**	1.93 **2.54**	1.87 **2.43**	1.82 **2.35**	1.78 **2.26**	1.72 **2.17**	1.69 **2.12**	1.65 **2.04**	1.62 **2.00**	1.59 **1.94**	1.56 **1.90**	1.55 **1.87**
38	4.10 **7.35**	3.25 **5.21**	2.85 **4.34**	2.62 **3.86**	2.46 **3.54**	2.35 **3.32**	2.26 **3.15**	2.19 **3.02**	2.14 **2.91**	2.09 **2.82**	2.05 **2.75**	2.02 **2.69**	1.96 **2.59**	1.92 **2.51**	1.85 **2.40**	1.80 **2.32**	1.76 **2.22**	1.71 **2.14**	1.67 **2.08**	1.63 **2.00**	1.60 **1.97**	1.57 **1.90**	1.54 **1.86**	1.53 **1.84**
40	4.08 **7.31**	3.23 **5.18**	2.84 **4.31**	2.61 **3.83**	2.45 **3.51**	2.34 **3.29**	2.25 **3.12**	2.18 **2.99**	2.12 **2.88**	2.07 **2.80**	2.04 **2.73**	2.00 **2.66**	1.95 **2.56**	1.90 **2.49**	1.84 **2.37**	1.79 **2.29**	1.74 **2.20**	1.69 **2.11**	1.66 **2.05**	1.61 **1.97**	1.59 **1.94**	1.55 **1.88**	1.53 **1.84**	1.51 **1.81**

(continued)

TABLE A.2 Critical Values of F Corresponding to p<.05 and p<.01 (Continued)

ν_n

ν_d	1	2	3	4	5	6	7	8	9	10	11	12	14	16	20	24	30	40	50	75	100	200	500	x
42	4.07 / **7.27**	3.22 / **5.15**	2.83 / **4.29**	2.59 / **3.80**	2.44 / **3.49**	2.32 / **3.26**	2.24 / **3.10**	2.17 / **2.96**	2.11 / **2.86**	2.06 / **2.77**	2.02 / **2.70**	1.99 / **2.64**	1.94 / **2.54**	1.89 / **2.46**	1.82 / **2.35**	1.78 / **2.26**	1.73 / **2.17**	1.68 / **2.08**	1.64 / **2.02**	1.60 / **1.94**	1.57 / **1.91**	1.54 / **1.85**	1.51 / **1.80**	1.49 / **1.78**
44	4.06 / **7.24**	3.21 / **5.12**	2.82 / **4.26**	2.58 / **3.78**	2.43 / **3.46**	2.31 / **3.24**	2.23 / **3.07**	2.16 / **2.94**	2.10 / **2.84**	2.05 / **2.75**	2.01 / **2.68**	1.98 / **2.62**	1.92 / **2.52**	1.88 / **2.44**	1.81 / **2.32**	1.76 / **2.24**	1.72 / **2.15**	1.66 / **2.06**	1.63 / **2.00**	1.58 / **1.92**	1.56 / **1.88**	1.52 / **1.82**	1.50 / **1.78**	1.48 / **1.75**
46	4.05 / **7.21**	3.20 / **5.10**	2.81 / **4.24**	2.57 / **3.76**	2.42 / **3.44**	2.30 / **3.22**	2.22 / **3.05**	2.14 / **2.92**	2.09 / **2.82**	2.04 / **2.73**	2.00 / **2.66**	1.97 / **2.60**	1.91 / **2.50**	1.87 / **2.42**	1.80 / **2.30**	1.75 / **2.22**	1.71 / **2.13**	1.65 / **2.04**	1.62 / **1.98**	1.57 / **1.90**	1.54 / **1.86**	1.51 / **1.80**	1.48 / **1.76**	1.46 / **1.72**
48	4.04 / **7.19**	3.19 / **5.08**	2.80 / **4.22**	2.56 / **3.74**	2.41 / **3.42**	2.30 / **3.20**	2.21 / **3.04**	2.14 / **2.90**	2.08 / **2.80**	2.03 / **2.71**	1.99 / **2.64**	1.96 / **2.58**	1.90 / **2.48**	1.86 / **2.40**	1.79 / **2.28**	1.74 / **2.20**	1.70 / **2.11**	1.64 / **2.02**	1.61 / **1.96**	1.56 / **1.88**	1.53 / **1.84**	1.50 / **1.78**	1.47 / **1.73**	1.45 / **1.70**
50	4.03 / **7.17**	3.18 / **5.06**	2.79 / **4.20**	2.56 / **3.72**	2.40 / **3.41**	2.29 / **3.18**	2.20 / **3.02**	2.13 / **2.88**	2.07 / **2.78**	2.02 / **2.70**	1.98 / **2.62**	1.95 / **2.56**	1.90 / **2.46**	1.85 / **2.39**	1.78 / **2.26**	1.74 / **2.18**	1.69 / **2.10**	1.63 / **2.00**	1.60 / **1.94**	1.55 / **1.86**	1.52 / **1.82**	1.48 / **1.76**	1.46 / **1.71**	1.44 / **1.68**
60	4.00 / **7.08**	3.15 / **4.98**	2.76 / **4.13**	2.52 / **3.65**	2.37 / **3.34**	2.25 / **3.12**	2.17 / **2.95**	2.10 / **2.82**	2.04 / **2.72**	1.99 / **2.63**	1.95 / **2.56**	1.92 / **2.50**	1.86 / **2.40**	1.81 / **2.32**	1.75 / **2.20**	1.70 / **2.12**	1.65 / **2.03**	1.59 / **1.93**	1.56 / **1.87**	1.50 / **1.79**	1.48 / **1.74**	1.44 / **1.68**	1.41 / **1.63**	1.39 / **1.60**
70	3.98 / **7.01**	3.13 / **4.92**	2.74 / **4.08**	2.50 / **3.60**	2.35 / **3.29**	2.23 / **3.07**	2.14 / **2.91**	2.07 / **2.77**	2.01 / **2.67**	1.97 / **2.59**	1.93 / **2.51**	1.89 / **2.45**	1.84 / **2.35**	1.79 / **2.28**	1.72 / **2.15**	1.67 / **2.07**	1.62 / **1.98**	1.56 / **1.88**	1.53 / **1.82**	1.47 / **1.74**	1.45 / **1.69**	1.40 / **1.62**	1.37 / **1.56**	1.35 / **1.53**
80	3.96 / **6.96**	3.11 / **4.88**	2.72 / **4.04**	2.48 / **3.56**	2.33 / **3.25**	2.21 / **3.04**	2.12 / **2.87**	2.05 / **2.74**	1.99 / **2.64**	1.95 / **2.55**	1.91 / **2.48**	1.88 / **2.41**	1.82 / **2.32**	1.77 / **2.24**	1.70 / **2.11**	1.65 / **2.03**	1.60 / **1.94**	1.54 / **1.84**	1.51 / **1.78**	1.45 / **1.70**	1.42 / **1.65**	1.38 / **1.57**	1.35 / **1.52**	1.32 / **1.49**
100	3.94 / **6.90**	3.09 / **4.82**	2.70 / **3.98**	2.46 / **3.51**	2.30 / **3.20**	2.19 / **2.99**	2.10 / **2.82**	2.03 / **2.69**	1.97 / **2.59**	1.92 / **2.51**	1.88 / **2.43**	1.85 / **2.36**	1.79 / **2.26**	1.75 / **2.19**	1.68 / **2.06**	1.63 / **1.98**	1.57 / **1.89**	1.51 / **1.79**	1.48 / **1.73**	1.42 / **1.64**	1.39 / **1.59**	1.34 / **1.51**	1.30 / **1.46**	1.28 / **1.43**
120	3.92 / **6.85**	3.07 / **4.79**	2.68 / **3.95**	2.45 / **3.48**	2.29 / **3.17**	2.18 / **2.96**	2.09 / **2.79**	2.02 / **2.66**	1.96 / **2.56**	1.91 / **2.47**	1.87 / **2.40**	1.84 / **2.34**	1.78 / **2.23**	1.73 / **2.15**	1.66 / **2.03**	1.61 / **1.95**	1.56 / **1.86**	1.50 / **1.76**	1.46 / **1.70**	1.39 / **1.61**	1.37 / **1.56**	1.32 / **1.48**	1.28 / **1.42**	1.25 / **1.38**
∞	3.84 / **6.63**	2.99 / **4.60**	2.60 / **3.78**	2.37 / **3.32**	2.21 / **3.02**	2.09 / **2.80**	2.01 / **2.64**	1.94 / **2.51**	1.88 / **2.41**	1.83 / **2.32**	1.79 / **2.24**	1.75 / **2.18**	1.69 / **2.07**	1.64 / **1.99**	1.57 / **1.87**	1.52 / **1.79**	1.46 / **1.69**	1.40 / **1.59**	1.35 / **1.52**	1.28 / **1.41**	1.24 / **1.36**	1.17 / **1.25**	1.11 / **1.15**	1.00 / **1.00**

Lightface values correspond to $p < 0.05$ and boldface values correspond to $p < 0.01$.

ν_n, degrees of freedom for numerator; ν_d, degrees of freedom for denominator.

Reproduced from Glantz SA. Primer of Biostatistics (6th ed.), New York: McGraw-Hill; 2005. Table 3-1. Critical values of F corresponding to p < .05 (Lightface) and p < .01 (Boldface). PP. 52–54, with permission from McGraw-Hill and original source: Adapted from G. W. Snedecor and W. G. Cochran, Statistical Methods. Iowa State University Press. Ames 1978, pp. 560–563.

TABLE A.3   Critical Values of *t* (Two-Tailed)

ν	\multicolumn{9}{c}{Probability of greater value, P}
	0.50	0.20	0.10	0.05	0.02	0.01	0.005	0.002	0.001
1	1.000	3.078	6.314	12.706	31.821	63.657	127.321	318.309	636.619
2	0.816	1.886	2.920	4.303	6.965	9.925	14.089	22.327	31.599
3	0.765	1.638	2.353	3.182	4.541	5.841	7.453	10.215	12.924
4	0.741	1.533	2.132	2.776	3.747	4.604	5.598	7.173	8.610
5	0.727	1.476	2.015	2.571	3.365	4.032	4.773	5.893	6.869
6	0.718	1.440	1.943	2.447	3.143	3.707	4.317	5.208	5.959
7	0.711	1.415	1.895	2.365	2.998	3.499	4.029	4.785	5.408
8	0.706	1.397	1.860	2.306	2.896	3.355	3.833	4.501	5.041
9	0.703	1.383	1.833	2.262	2.821	3.250	3.690	4.297	4.781
10	0.700	1.372	1.812	2.228	2.764	3.169	3.581	4.144	4.587
11	0.697	1.363	1.796	2.201	2.718	3.106	3.497	4.025	4.437
12	0.695	1.356	1.782	2.179	2.681	3.055	3.428	3.930	4.318
13	0.694	1.350	1.771	2.160	2.650	3.012	3.372	3.852	4.221
14	0.692	1.345	1.761	2.145	2.624	2.977	3.326	3.787	4.140
15	0.691	1.341	1.753	2.131	2.602	2.947	3.286	3.733	4.073
16	0.690	1.337	1.746	2.120	2.583	2.921	3.252	3.686	4.015
17	0.689	1.333	1.740	2.110	2.567	2.898	3.222	3.646	3.965
18	0.688	1.330	1.734	2.101	2.552	2.878	3.197	3.610	3.922
19	0.688	1.328	1.729	2.093	2.539	2.861	3.174	3.579	3.883
20	0.687	1.325	1.725	2.086	2.528	2.845	3.153	3.552	3.850
21	0.686	1.323	1.721	2.080	2.518	2.831	3.135	3.527	3.819
22	0.686	1.321	1.717	2.074	2.508	2.819	3.119	3.505	3.792
23	0.685	1.319	1.714	2.069	2.500	2.807	3.104	3.485	3.768
24	0.685	1.318	1.711	2.064	2.492	2.797	3.091	3.467	3.745
25	0.684	1.316	1.708	2.060	2.485	2.787	3.078	3.450	3.725
26	0.684	1.315	1.706	2.056	2.479	2.779	3.067	3.435	3.707
27	0.684	1.314	1.703	2.052	2.473	2.771	3.057	3.421	3.690
28	0.683	1.313	1.701	2.048	2.467	2.763	3.047	3.408	3.674
29	0.683	1.311	1.699	2.045	2.462	2.756	3.038	3.396	3.659
30	0.683	1.310	1.697	2.042	2.457	2.750	3.030	3.385	3.646
31	0.682	1.309	1.696	2.040	2.453	2.744	3.022	3.375	3.633
32	0.682	1.309	1.694	2.037	2.449	2.738	3.015	3.365	3.622
33	0.682	1.308	1.692	2.035	2.445	2.733	3.008	3.356	3.611
34	0.682	1.307	1.691	2.032	2.441	2.728	3.002	3.348	3.601
35	0.682	1.306	1.690	2.030	2.438	2.724	2.996	3.340	3.591
36	0.981	1.306	1.688	2.028	2.434	2.719	2.990	3.333	3.582
37	0.681	1.305	1.687	20.26	2.431	2.715	2.985	3.326	3.574
38	0.681	1.304	1.686	2.024	2.429	2.712	2.980	3.319	3.566
39	0.681	1.304	1.685	2.023	2.426	2.708	2.976	3.313	3.558
40	0.681	1.303	1.684	2.021	2.423	2.704	2.971	3.307	3.551

(continued)

TABLE A.3   Critical Values of t (Two-Tailed) (*Continued*)

				Probability of greater value, P					
ν	0.50	0.20	0.10	0.05	0.02	0.01	0.005	0.002	0.001
42	0.680	1.302	1.682	2.018	2.418	2.698	2.963	3.296	3.538
44	0.680	1.301	1.680	2.015	2.414	2.692	2.956	3.286	3.526
46	0.680	1.300	1.679	2.013	2.410	2.687	2.949	3.277	3.515
48	0.680	1.299	1.677	2.011	2.407	2.682	2.943	3.269	3.505
50	0.679	1.299	1.676	2.009	2.403	2.678	2.937	3.261	3.496
52	0.679	1.298	1.675	2.007	2.400	2.674	2.932	3.255	3.488
54	0.679	1.297	1.674	2.005	2.397	2.670	2.927	3.248	3.480
56	0.679	1.297	1.673	2.003	2.395	2.667	2.923	3.242	3.473
58	0.679	1.296	1.672	2.002	2.392	2.663	2.918	3.237	3.466
60	0.679	1.296	1.671	2.000	2.390	2.660	2.915	3.232	3.460
62	0.678	1.295	1.670	1.999	2.388	2.657	2.911	3.227	3.454
64	0.678	1.295	1.669	1.998	2.386	2.655	2.908	3.223	3.449
66	0.678	1.295	1.668	1.997	2.384	2.652	2.904	3.218	3.444
68	0.678	1.294	1.668	1.995	2.382	2.650	2.902	3.214	3.439
70	0.678	1.294	1.667	1.994	2.381	2.648	2.899	3.211	3.435
72	0.678	1.293	1.666	1.993	2.379	2.646	2.896	3.207	3.431
74	0.678	1.293	1.666	1.993	2.378	2.644	2.894	3.204	3.427
76	0.678	1.293	1.665	1.992	2.376	2.642	2.891	3.201	3.423
78	0.678	1.292	1.665	1.991	2.375	2.640	2.889	3.198	3.420
80	0.678	1.292	1.664	1.990	2.374	2.639	2.887	3.195	3.416
90	0.677	1.291	1.662	1.987	2.368	2.632	2.878	3.183	3.402
100	0.677	1.290	1.660	1.984	2.364	2.626	2.871	3.174	3.390
120	0.677	1.289	1.658	1.980	2.358	2.617	2.860	3.160	3.373
140	0.676	1.288	1.656	1.977	2.353	2.611	2.852	3.149	3.361
160	0.676	1.287	1.654	1.975	2.350	2.607	2.846	3.142	3.352
180	0.676	1.286	1.653	1.973	2.347	2.603	2.842	3.136	3.345
200	0.676	1.286	1.653	1.972	2.345	2.601	2.839	3.131	3.340
∞	0.6745	1.2816	1.6449	1.9600	2.3263	2.5758	2.8070	3.0902	3.2905

Reproduced from Glantz SA. Primer of Biostatistics (6th ed.), New York: McGraw-Hill; 2005. Table 4-1. Critical Values of t (Two-Tailed). pp. 90–91, with permission from McGraw-Hill and original source: Adapted from J. H. Zar, Biostatistical Analysis (2nd ed.), Prentice-Hall, Englewood Cliffs, N.J., 1984, pp. 484–485, Table B.3.

TABLE A.4   Critical Values for the χ^2 (Distribution)

	Probability of greater value, P							
ν	.50	.25	.10	.05	.025	.01	.005	.001
1	.455	1.323	2.706	3.841	5.024	6.635	7.879	10.828
2	1.386	2.773	4.605	5.991	7.378	9.210	10.597	13.816
3	2.366	4.108	6.251	7.815	9.348	11.345	12.838	16.266
4	3.357	5.385	7.779	9.488	11.143	13.277	14.860	18.467
5	4.351	6.626	9.236	11.070	12.833	15.086	16.750	20.515
6	5.348	7.841	10.645	12.592	14.449	16.812	18.548	22.458
7	6.346	9.037	12.017	14.067	16.013	18.475	20.278	24.322
8	7.344	10.219	13.362	15.507	17.535	20.090	21.955	26.124
9	8.343	11.389	14.684	16.919	19.023	21.666	23.589	27.877
10	9.342	12.549	15.987	18.307	20.483	23.209	25.188	29.588
11	10.341	13.701	17.275	19.675	21.920	24.725	26.757	31.264
12	11.340	14.845	18.549	21.026	23.337	26.217	28.300	32.909
13	12.340	15.984	19.812	22.362	24.736	27.688	29.819	34.528
14	13.339	17.117	21.064	23.685	26.119	29.141	31.319	36.123
15	14.339	18.245	22.307	24.996	27.488	30.578	32.801	37.697
16	15.338	19.369	23.542	26.296	28.845	32.000	34.267	39.252
17	16.338	20.489	24.769	27.587	30.191	33.409	35.718	40.790
18	17.338	21.605	25.989	28.869	31.526	34.805	37.156	42.312
19	18.338	22.718	27.204	30.144	32.852	36.191	38.582	43.820
20	19.337	23.828	28.412	31.410	34.170	37.566	39.997	45.315
21	20.337	24.935	29.615	32.671	35.479	38.932	41.401	46.797
22	21.337	26.039	30.813	33.924	36.781	40.289	42.796	48.268
23	22.337	27.141	32.007	35.172	38.076	41.638	44.181	49.728
24	23.337	28.241	33.196	36.415	39.364	42.980	45.559	51.179
25	24.337	29.339	34.382	37.652	40.646	44.314	46.928	52.620
26	25.336	30.435	35.563	38.885	41.923	45.642	48.290	54.052
27	26.336	31.528	36.741	40.113	43.195	46.963	49.645	55.476
28	27.336	32.020	37.916	41.337	44.461	48.278	50.993	56.892
29	28.336	33.711	39.087	42.557	45.722	49.588	52.336	58.301
30	29.336	34.800	40.256	43.773	46.979	50.892	53.672	59.703
31	30.336	35.887	41.422	44.985	48.232	52.191	55.003	61.098
32	31.336	36.973	42.585	46.194	49.480	53.486	56.328	62.487
33	32.336	38.058	43.745	47.400	50.725	54.776	57.648	63.870
34	33.336	39.141	44.903	48.602	51.966	56.061	58.964	65.247
35	34.336	40.223	46.059	49.802	53.203	57.342	60.275	66.619
36	35.336	41.304	47.212	50.998	54.437	58.619	61.581	67.985
37	36.336	42.383	48.363	52.192	55.668	59.893	62.883	69.346
38	37.335	43.462	49.513	53.384	56.896	61.162	64.181	70.703
39	38.335	44.539	50.660	54.572	58.120	62.428	65.476	72.055
40	39.335	45.616	51.805	55.758	59.342	63.691	66.766	73.402

(continued)

TABLE A.4   Critical Values for the χ^2 (Distribution) (*Continued*)

ν	Probability of greater value, *P*							
	.50	**.25**	**.10**	**.05**	**.025**	**.01**	**.005**	**.001**
41	40.335	46.692	52.949	56.942	60.561	64.950	68.053	74.745
42	41.335	47.766	54.090	58.124	61.777	66.206	69.336	76.084
43	42.335	48.840	55.230	59.304	62.990	67.459	70.616	77.419
44	43.335	49.913	56.369	60.481	64.201	68.710	71.893	78.750
45	44.335	50.985	57.505	61.656	65.410	69.957	73.166	80.077
46	45.335	52.056	58.641	62.830	66.617	71.201	74.437	81.400
47	46.335	53.127	59.774	64.001	67.821	72.443	75.704	82.720
48	47.335	54.196	60.907	65.171	69.023	73.683	76.969	84.037
49	48.335	55.265	62.038	66.339	70.222	74.919	78.231	85.351
50	49.335	56.334	63.167	67.505	71.420	76.154	79.490	86.661

Reproduced from Glantz SA. Primer of Biostatistics. (6th ed.), New York: McGraw-Hill;
2005. Table 5-7. Critical Values for the χ^2 Distribution. pp. 156–157, with permission
from McGraw-Hill and original source: Adapted from J. H. Zar, Biostatistical Analysis
(2nd ed.) Prentice-Hall, Englewood Cliffs, N.J. 1984, pp. 479–482, Table B.1.

TABLE A.5   Critical Values (Two-Tailed) of the Mann-Whitney Rank-Sum Statistic T

		Probability levels near			
		.05		**.01**	
n_s	n_b	**Critical values**	**P**	**Critical values**	**P**
3	4	6,18	.057		
	5	6,21	.036		
	5	7,20	.071		
	6	7,23	.048	6,24	.024
	7	7,26	.033	6,27	.017
	7	8,25	.067		
	8	8,28	.042	6,30	.012
4	4	11,25	.057	10,26	.026
	5	11,29	.032	10,30	.016
	5	12,28	.063		
	6	12,32	.038	10,34	.010
	7	13,35	.042	10,38	.012
	8	14,38	.048	11,41	.008
	8	....	....	12,40	.016
5	5	17,38	.032	15,40	.008
	5	18,37	.056	16,39	.016
	6	19,41	.052	16,44	.010
	7	20,45	.048	17,48	.010
	8	21,49	.045	18,52	.011
6	6	26,52	.041	23,55	.009
	6	....	....	24,54	.015
	7	28,56	.051	24,60	.008
	7	....	....	25,59	.014
	8	29,61	.043	25,65	.008
	8	30,60	.059	26,64	.013
7	7	37,68	.053	33,72	.011
	8	39,73	.054	34,78	.009
8	8	49,87	.050	44,92	.010

Reproduced from Glantz SA. Primer of Biostatistics (6th ed.), New York: McGraw-Hill; 2005. Table 10-3. Critical Values (Two-Tailed) of the Mann-Whitney Rank-Sum Statistic T. pp. 371, with permission from McGraw-Hill and original source: Computed from F. Mosteller and R. Rourke, Sturdy Statistics: Non-parametrics and Order Statistics, Addison-Wesley, Reading, MA, 1973, Table A-9.

TABLE A.6   Critical Values (Two-Tailed) of Wilcoxon W

n	Critical value	P	n	Critical value	P
5	15	.062	13	65	.022
6	21	.032		57	.048
	19	.062	14	73	.020
7	28	.016		63	.050
	24	.046	15	80	.022
8	32	.024		70	.048
	28	.054	16	88	.020
9	39	.020		76	.050
	33	.054	17	97	.020
10	45	.020		83	.050
	39	.048	18	105	.020
11	52	.018		91	.048
	44	.054	19	114	.020
12	58	.020		98	.050
	50	.052	20	124	.020
				106	.048

Reproduced from Glantz SA. Primer of Biostatistics (6th ed.), New York: McGraw-Hill; 2005. Table 10-7. Critical Values (Two-Tails) of Wilcoxon W. pp. 383, with permission from McGraw-Hill and original source: Adapted from F. Mostelle; and R. Rourke, Sturdy Statistics: Non-parametrics and Order Statistics, Addison-Wesley, Reading. MA, 1973, Table A-11.

TABLE A.7   Critical Values for Spearman Rank Correlation Coefficient*

n	.50	.20	.10	.05	.02	.01	.005	.002	.001
				Probability of greater value, P					
4	.600	1.000	1.000						
5	.500	.800	.900	1.000	1.000				
6	.371	.657	.829	.886	.943	1.000	1.000		
7	.321	.571	.714	.786	.893	.929	.964	1.000	1.000
8	.310	.524	.643	.738	.833	.881	.905	.952	.976
9	.267	.483	.600	.700	.783	.833	.867	.917	.933
10	.248	.455	.564	.648	.745	.794	.830	.879	.903
11	.236	.427	.536	.618	.709	.755	.800	.845	.873
12	.217	.406	.503	.587	.678	.727	.769	.818	.846
13	.209	.385	.484	.560	.648	.703	.747	.791	.824
14	.200	.367	.464	.538	.626	.679	.723	.771	.802
15	.189	.354	.446	.521	.604	.654	.700	.750	.779
16	.182	.341	.429	.503	.582	.635	.679	.729	.762
17	.176	.328	.414	.485	.566	.615	.662	.713	.748
18	.170	.317	.401	.472	.550	.600	.643	.695	.728
19	.165	.309	.391	.460	.535	.584	.628	.677	.712
20	.161	.299	.380	.447	.520	.570	.612	.662	.696
21	.156	.292	.370	.435	.508	.556	.599	.648	.681
22	.152	.284	.361	.425	.496	.544	.586	.634	.667
23	.148	.278	.353	.415	.486	.532	.573	.622	.654
24	.144	.271	.344	.406	.476	.521	.562	.610	.642
25	.142	.265	.337	.398	.466	.511	.551	.598	.630
26	.138	.259	.331	.390	.457	.501	.541	.587	.619
27	.136	.255	.324	.382	.448	.491	.531	.577	.608
28	.133	.250	.317	.375	.440	.483	.522	.567	.598
29	.130	.245	.312	.368	.433	.475	.513	.558	.589
30	.128	.240	.306	.362	.425	.467	.504	.549	.580
31	.126	.236	.301	.356	.418	.459	.496	.541	.571
32	.124	.232	.296	.350	.412	.452	.489	.533	.563
33	.121	.229	.291	.345	.405	.446	.482	.525	.554
34	.120	.225	.287	.340	.399	.439	.475	.517	.547
35	.118	.222	.283	.335	.394	.433	.468	.510	.539
36	.116	.219	.279	.330	.388	.427	.462	.504	.533
37	.114	.216	.275	.325	.383	.421	.456	.497	.526
38	.113	.212	.271	.321	.378	.415	.450	.491	.519
39	.111	.210	.267	.317	.373	.410	.444	.485	.513
40	.110	.207	.264	.313	.368	.405	.439	.479	.507

(continued)

TABLE A.7   Critical Values for Spearman Rank Correlation Coefficient* (*Continued*)

	Probability of greater value, P								
n	.50	.20	.10	.05	.02	.01	.005	.002	.001
41	.108	.204	.261	.309	.364	.400	.433	.473	.501
42	.107	.202	.257	.305	.359	.395	.428	.468	.495
43	.105	.199	.254	.301	.355	.391	.423	.463	.490
44	.104	.197	.251	.298	.351	.386	.419	.458	.484
45	.103	.194	.248	.294	.347	.382	.414	.453	.479
46	.102	.192	.246	.291	.343	.378	.410	.448	.474
47	.101	.190	.243	.288	.340	.374	.405	.443	.469
48	.100	.188	.240	.285	.336	.370	.401	.439	.465
49	.098	.186	.238	.282	.333	.366	.497	.434	.460
50	.097	.184	.235	.279	.329	.363	.393	.430	.456

*For sample sizes greater than 50, use $t = \dfrac{r_s}{\sqrt{(1 - r_s^2)/(n-2)}}$
with $v = n - 2$ degrees of freedom to obtain the approximate p value.

Reproduced from Glantz SA. Primer of Biostatistics (6th ed.), New York: McGraw-Hill; 2005. Table 8-6. Critical values for Spearman rank correlation coefficient. pp. 298–299, with permission from McGraw-Hill and original source: Adapted from J. H. Zar, Biostatistical Analysis (2nd ed.), Prentice-Hall, Englewood Cliffs, N.J. 1974, pp. 498.

Annotated
Bibliography

The sources, as given next, have been selected either to reinforce concepts covered in this text or to provide additional, more advanced information for those who wish to learn more about specific topics.

Chapter 2

1. Glantz SA. Primer of Biostatistics (6th ed.), New York: McGraw-Hill; 2005. *Basic descriptive statistics is covered nicely in Chapter 2. Analysis of variance and the t test are covered in Chapters 3 and 4, respectively. Nice coverage on methods based on ranks is given in Chapter 10.*

2. University of Edinburgh. Chi-squared test for categories of data. Available from: www.helios.bto.ed.ac.uk/bto/statistics/tress9.html. *Nice web-based summary of the χ^2 test is given here.*

3. Bower KM. When to use Fisher's exact test. Available from: www.minitab.com/resources/articles/FisherExact.pdf. *Good explanation of Fisher's exact test with simple example is given here.*

4. Zou KH, Tuncali K, Silverman SG. Correlation and simple linear regression. Radiology 2003;227:617–628. *This reference includes a nice example from the field of radiology.*

Chapter 3

1. Elstein AS, Schwarz A. Clinical problem solving and diagnostic decision making: Selective review of the cognitive literature. BMJ 2002; 324(733). *An overview of how doctors think about diagnosis is given here.*

2. Sox HC, Blatt MA, Higgins MC, Marton KI. *Medical Decision Making.* Boston, MA: Butterworths; 1988. *Chapters 2 and 4, entitled Differential Diagnosis and Understanding New Information: Bayes' Theorem, respectively, provide more information about the psychology of diagnostic reasoning and review basic concepts such as conditional probability.*

Chapter 4

1. Everitt BS, Pickles A. Statistical aspects of the design and analysis of clinical trials. London: Imperial College Press; 1999. *This is a fantastic book! Chapter 2, entitled Treatment Allocation, the Size of Trials and*

Reporting Results, is easy to read and covers important principles of random-ization and sample size determination.

2. Beller EM, Glebski V, Keech AC. Randomisation in clinical trials. MJA 2002;177:565–567. *It is a nice short article about different approaches to randomization.*

3. van Belle G. Statistical rules of thumb. Available from: www.vanbelle. org/toc.htm. *Dr. Van Belle's freely accessible online textbook includes Chapter 2, Sample Size, which is especially useful.*

Chapter 5

1. Sterne JAC, Smith GD. Sifting the evidence—what's wrong with signif-icance tests. BMJ 2001;322:226–231. *This provides a nice overview of limi-tations of p values and significance tests.*

2. Goodman SN. Toward evidence-based medical statistics. 1: The p value fallacy. Ann Intern Med 1999;130:995–1004. *It is the first of two arti-cles by Dr. Goodman, which makes a convincing case for an alternative to p values.*

3. Goodman SN. Toward evidence-based medical statistics. 2: The Bayes factor. Ann Intern Med 1999;130:1005–1013. *There is a description of the alternative Bayesian approach to interpretation of the results of clinical trials.*

4. Greenfield MLVH, Kuhn JE, Wojtys EM. A statistics primer. Confidence intervals. Am J Sports Med 1998;26(1):145–149. *Basic description of CIs and their importance is given here.*

Chapter 6

1. Centers for Disease Control. Epidemiology Program Office. Case stud-ies in applied epidemiology. Cigarette smoking and lung cancer. Avail-able from: www.cdc.gov/eis/casestudies/xsmoke.student.731-703.pdf. *This is a very useful set of exercises that illustrates the cohort and case control designs as well as ORs.*

2. Alfeld P. What on earth is a logarithm? Available from: www.math. utah.edu/~pa/math/log.html. *It is a nice, simple review of logarithms to reinforce the brief review that appears in this chapter.*

Chapter 7

1. Bull K, Spiegelhalter DJ. Tutorial in biostatistics. Survival analysis in observational studies. Stat Med 1997;16:1041–1074. *It is a nicely writ-ten article that covers a number of key concepts including censoring, the*

Kaplan-Meier method, the logrank test, and Cox proportional hazards survival analysis.

2. Clark TG, Bradburn MJ, Love SB, Altman DG. Survival analysis part I: Basic concepts and first analyses. Br J Cancer 2003;89:232–238. *This is the first article in a series of four excellent articles about survival analysis, which includes several advanced topics. Sources for the remaining three articles are listed next.*

3. Bradburn MJ, Clark TG, Love SB, Altman DG. Survival analysis part II: Multivariate data analysis—an introduction to concepts and methods. Br J Cancer 2003;89:431–436.

4. Bradburn MJ, Clark TG, Love SB, Altman DG. Survival analysis part III: Multivariate data analysis—choosing a model and assessing its adequacy and fit. Br J Cancer 2003;89:605–611.

5. Clark TG, Bradburn MJ, Love SB, Altman DG. Survival analysis part IV: Further concepts and methods in survival analysis. Br J Cancer 2003;89:781–786.

Chapter 8

1. Cochrane Collaboration. Cochrane handbook for systematic reviews of interventions. Available from: www.cochrane.dk/cochrane/handbook/hbook.htm. *The Cochrane Collaboration is the world's leading organization dedicated to producing high-quality systematic reviews. The precise methods through which reviews are produced are described in the handbook.*

2. Jackson J. Meta-analysis. Available from: www.sgim.org/AM03Handouts/PA04.pdf. *This is a handout from a 2003 conference that is freely available on the Internet. Dr. Jackson provides an excellent overview of the procedures used in meta-analysis.*

3. DerSimonian R, Laird N. Meta-analysis in clinical trials. Contr Clin Trials 1986;7:177–188. *Description of a commonly used random effects method for pooling results for a meta-analysis is given here.*

4. Higgins JPT, Thompson SG, Deeks JJ, Altman DG. Measuring inconsistency in meta-analysis. BMJ 2003;327:557–560. *The article introduces the concept of inconsistency as an alternative to Cochran's Q.*

Chapter 9

1. Detsky AS, Naglie G, Krahn MD, Naimark D, Redelmeier DA. Primer on medical decision analysis: Part 1—Getting started. Med Decis

Making 1997;17:123–125. *This is the first of a five-part series of articles that covers the breadth of decision analysis. Although 10 years old, these articles still represent an excellent tutorial. The remaining four articles in the series are listed next.*

2. Detsky AS, Naglie G, Krahn MD, Redelmeier DA, Naimark D. Primer on medical decision analysis: Part 2—Building a tree. Med Decis Making 1997;17:126–135.

3. Naglie G, Krahn MD, Naimark D, Redelmeier DA, Detsky AS. Primer on medical decision analysis: Part 3—Estimating probabilities and utilities. Med Decis Making 1997;17:136–141.

4. Krahn MD, Naglie G, Naimark D, Redelmeier DA, Detsky AS. Primer on medical decision analysis: Part 4—Analyzing the model and interpreting the results. Med Decis Making 1997;17:142–151.

5. Naimark D, Krahn MD, Naglie G, Redelmeier DA, Detsky AS. Primer on medical decision analysis: Part 5—Working with Markov processes. Med Decis Making 1997;17:152–159.

6. Sox HC, Blatt MA, Higgins MC, Marton KI. *Medical Decision Making.* Boston, MA: Butterworths; 1988. *Chapters 6 and 7, entitled Expected Value Decision Making and Measuring the Outcome of Care, provide an excellent overview of simple decision analysis and assessment of utility. Chapter 11 provides an introduction to cost-effectiveness and cost-benefit analysis.*

Chapter 10

1. Kish MA. Guide to development of practice guidelines. Clin Infect Dis 2001;32:851–854. *A nice, brief description of how guidelines are developed has been provided.*

2. Turoff M, Linstone HA, eds. The Delphi method: Techniques and applications. Available from: www.is.njit.edu/pubs/delphibook/. *It is a freely available online textbook for those who wish to learn more about the Delphi method.*

Index